Behind the Screens
Nursing, Somology, and the
Problem of the Body

Jocalyn Lawler RN PhD FRCNA FCN (NSW)

Associate Professor of Nursing,
University of New England,
Armidale, New South Wales

CHURCHILL LIVINGSTONE
MELBOURNE EDINBURGH LONDON NEW YORK AND TOKYO 1991

CHURCHILL LIVINGSTONE
Medical Division of Longman Group UK Limited

Distributed in Australia by Longman Cheshire Pty Limited,
Longman House, Kings Gardens, 95 Coventry Street, South
Melbourne 3205, and distributed throughout the world, with
the exception of Canada and the United States of America,
by associated companies, branches and representatives.

First published 1991

ISBN 0-443-04444-9

British Library Cataloguing in Publication Data
Lawler, Jocalyn
    Behind the screens: nursing, somology and the problem of
    the body.
    1. Medicine. Nursing
    I. Title
    610.73

Library of Congress Cataloging in Publication Data
Lawler, Jocalyn.
    Behind the screens: nursing, somology, and the problem
    of the body/Jocalyn Lawler.
    p. cm.
    Includes bibliographical references.
    Includes index.
    ISBN 0-443-04444-9
    1. Nurse and patient. 2. Somesthesia.
    3. Nurses — Attitudes. 4. Nursing — Psychological
    aspects. I. Title.
    [DNLM: 1. Body Image. 2. Kinesics.
    3. Nurses — psychology. 4. Nursing.   WY 87 L418b]
RT86.3.L39   1991
610. 73 — dc20
DNLM/DLC
for Library of Congress

Produced by Longman Singapore Publisher's Pte Ltd
Printed in Singapore

Preface

When I first began this research for a PhD in sociology in 1985 few people were publicly interested in the issues which are explored here, and I became aware very early in the project that I was researching areas on the fringe of respectability. My original supervisor, Terry Leahy, helped me to believe that it was possible to study taboo topics such as excreta, genitalia, and dirty work, and furthermore, that it was important to do so. He provided the intellectual climate which allowed my ideas to take shape according to what my experience as a nurse and the literature told me. Without his assistance I may not have persisted with this area of research. I am pleased I did because I am finding it increasingly fascinating and increasingly topical in nursing and sociology.

I had originally started this project with a vague idea about studying why it is that nurses are so often ignored and taken for granted. As a feminist I had an enduring interest in nursing as women's work, but the more I looked for answers the less I was satisfied with the notion of women's work as the only possible explanation for nurses' invisibility. I looked also for some guidance in the literature on dirty work, but this did not add a great deal, though it was interesting and useful. In my search for a way of explaining the relative invisibility of nursing care, I kept returning to the notion that some of what nurses did as work was regarded as highly private and it tended, in general conversation, to make people socially uncomfortable. The central notion in all this, when I eventually saw it, was both the presence of the body and the relative absence of any discourse on the body. I therefore came to study the body in nursing more by accident than design. That I stumbled across it, so to speak, is indicative of how taken-for-granted the body is in our everyday lives.

When I eventually turned my attention to the body as my primary focus and the more I read and reflected, the more it seemed to me

body was the pivotal construct which had the capacity to
ain lots of things about nursing as an occupation. More than
nat, however, I came to realise that nursing practice is essentially
and fundamentally about people's experiences of embodied
existence, particularly at those times when the body fails to function
normally.

This research has left me with a very profound and new respect
for nurses. I have become deeply impressed with the extent of their
sensitivity to the experiences of their patients, and I have become
even more sceptical about what traditional logico-positivist science
offers an occupation such as nursing. The issues which are discussed
in this book cannot be reduced to categories of care or levels of
illness – they are too rich in both socially constructed meaning and
the situations which locate individual experiences in time and
space. To that end, I am even more convinced that what separates
the (proper) nurse from those who are technically competent to
perform nursing care is not *what* is done, but rather *how* it is done
– that is, nursing is more a social entity than anything else. I am
also more convinced than ever that the debate over whether nursing
is (or can be) a science, or an art, or some mixture is really no
argument at all. Nursing is none of these, though people are trying
to make it look scientific. I think we should get on with the business
of articulating what a rich and interesting discipline it is, and just
call it nursing.

Armidale, 1991   J. L.

Acknowledgements

I owe a great deal to the nurses who helped in this study, in particular Marianne Murphy, Rosemary McIndoe and Barbara Chapman who all generously organised some of the interviews for this study. Without their assistance my task would have been much more difficult.

The people who agreed to be interviewed require special mention. They not only gave their time freely, they also talked openly about many things which one does not often discuss except with trusted colleagues. I thank them for their trust and the information they provided. My only regret is that they cannot be identified and they will not therefore receive the recognition I think they deserve for their skills, their sensitivity, and their ability.

Lois Bryson, who took over my supervision in 1987, was exceptionally supportive, constructive, and encouraging while I wrote the many drafts which a thesis requires.

My thanks go also to Judy Waters who had a vision of what my study would look like as a book, and to Rhonda Nay for the title. Most thanks, however, go to Cheryl Cordery for her patience and support during the study.

J.L.

Key to transcripts

[   ] added to make the context and/or meaning clear

... words, phrases or sentences of the interview deleted

R. means the researcher

I. means the interviewee

Italics are used for interview material

Contents

Introduction

This book describes a study about the body and social life, about how the body is managed by nurses in their work in our culture, and about what I have called 'the problem of the body'. To the extent that the body and some of its functions have been constructed as private matters, it is a subject which is not readily researchable. Almost by definition, if a subject is taboo it is difficult if not impossible to research. I chose to use nurses' experiences as a 'window' to the body so that we might better understand how the body is constructed in social life and to find out more about the highly private and invisible parts of nurses' work.

In our society, the body has a fragmented, silent, and ambiguous presence despite an obvious and prominent fact about human beings: they have bodies and they are bodies. More lucidly, human beings are embodied, just as they are enselved. Our everyday life is dominated by the details of our corporeal existence, involving us in a constant labour of eating, washing, grooming, dressing and sleeping (Turner 1984:1).

As a registered nurse, I know that nurses' work brings them into sustained and intimate contact with people who need help with what Turner (1984:1) calls 'the details of . . . corporeal existence', and that most patients require some assistance with the body. In requiring and providing that assistance, patients and nurses must socially negotiate the various norms, values, taboos, beliefs, and learned ways of behaving with respect to the body, which need redefinition in the context of reduced individual independence. And they must socially accommodate the body as a physical and biological entity. In order to manage these aspects of life and nursing practice, nurses must first know about taken-for-granted rules which govern the body in social life, and about the ways in which their role as nurses is assigned a particular place in the social ordering of the body.

'The problem of the body' is a function of two things – the organisation of knowledges, and a way of life which has rendered the body private and silent. The emphasis on empiricism,[1] abstract knowledge and increasing specialisation in the sciences (and academia generally) have resulted in a theoretical and epistemological fragmentation of our corporeal and embodied existence. 'The problem of the body' means, therefore, that, although a social and human body is integral to our existence, no discipline has yet overtly, explicitly and theoretically accommodated it, except in pieces. The body has been subjected to reduction and so too has our knowledge and experience of the body in social life. Our understanding of the body has been constructed in terms of the separate body and mind and not one entity of body and mind.

The physical body is the subject matter of a number of disciplines, for example, biochemistry, physiology, pathology, and medicine. More recently, the body has become the focus of attention for new disciplines, such as ergonomics, kinesiology, and chiropractic, each of which takes a particular, specialised and usually scientific, view of the body. Although these disciplines, to a greater or lesser extent, take account of social factors, they share a common framework which is fundamentally mechanistic, reductive and empiricist, and they view the body as an objective reality. Such a viewpoint leaves little space for other aspects of lived existence, such as feelings and emotions, except to the extent that these things can be understood as biologically determined processes – albeit processes which can be influenced by social life.

As the physical body has been increasingly fragmented by the organisation of knowledges, so too have the mind and non-material aspects of being. Several disciplines, for example, psychology, education, neurology, sociology and psychiatry now concern one or other aspect of how we think or behave. Although these disciplines acknowledge physical being, they are nevertheless fundamentally concerned with social organisation, individual behaviour and group processes which leave little space for the body.

The organisation of knowledges, as we currently know it, pivots on differences and on methodologies which institutionalise those differences. One consequence of this process is that territorial boundaries are established and maintained between disciplines. Works which attempt to cross these boundaries do not cause a shift in the organisation of knowledges because such works are conceptualised as 'interdisciplinary' or 'multidisciplinary'. Questions which do not reflect the existing organisation of knowledges or dominant paradigms and methodologies are variously labelled 'non-scientific', 'applied', or 'practical', among other things – locating them beyond the margins of legitimate and mainstream scholarship.

Becoming an accredited knower of the world – an academic, a scientist, a scholar, a nurse – requires one to learn ways of seeing, ways of knowing, and ways of sharing that knowledge. That means operating within disciplinary boundaries and procedures established over the last two centuries in Europe and North America by upper-middle and upper class white men (Hubbard 1988:6).

More recently, however, feminism and the works of Foucault (1974a, 1974b) are beginning to challenge thinking about the construction of knowledges. Feminists have been particularly and generally critical of established disciplines and their boundaries, especially where they are sexist if not misogynist (see, for example, Oakley 1974, especially Ch. 1, Ashley 1980, Spender 1981, Strathern 1985, Harding 1986, Longino 1988, Haraway 1988, Keller 1988, Genova 1988, Caine et al 1988). These critiques raise questions about why certain boundaries exist between disciplines, what processes maintain them, what is admitted or excluded as legitimate knowledge and why; and they focus attention on the consequences of our construction of knowledges.

The study reported in this book is an attempt to illustrate that the existing disciplinary framework and reduction of knowledges will not accommodate the body in social life and that 'the problem of the body' is in part a consequence of a configuration of knowledges which excludes it. I will argue, however, that nursing can, and does, necessarily and inevitably accommodate the body and corporeal existence, but that, for various reasons, the body's presence in nursing literature has been implicit, subsumed and privatised. In nursing practice, though, the body is very explicit and known in a way which is integrative of mind and body and which emphasises embodied existence in everyday life. 'The problem of the body', however, is such that nurses' work presents them with some very real social difficulties both in practice and in social life and it presents theoretical difficulties for the discipline and its relationship to other disciplines.

This research is about those difficulties and about the ways that nurses deal with them, and it is an attempt to explicate the body by drawing on the experiences of nurses whose work involves helping others with the 'constant labour of eating, washing, grooming, dressing and sleeping' (Turner 1984:1). Nurses call this 'basic body care' but, in the context of a patriarchal society, it is work typical of the domain of women and it is classical women's work (see Finch & Groves 1983). What is reported here is, therefore, about nursing practice and work associated with the caring roles of women. It is also about aspects of corporeal and embodied existence which have been privatised and designated as dirty work in social life and which have therefore also been largely ignored in academia.

Existing explanatory frameworks and methodologies do not adequately accommodate the body within the social sciences, and neither has nursing yet accommodated it theoretically or methodologically, although there have been some attempts (Benner 1984, 1988, Parker 1988, Gadow 1980, 1982, Colliere 1986, Wolf 1986a, 1986b). Such attempts have not made the body their central and primary concern as I have done here, but they have contributed to a process which will, if it continues, acknowledge the body as a pivotal concern for the practice of nursing. However, nursing has been ambivalent about the body both with respect to ideologies and practice, and in putting ideologies into practice.

Nursing's discomfort with the body not only reflects prevailing attitudes, but it also reflects a construction of knowledges and an emphasis on empiricism which do not make a space for the body. This study is an attempt to make such a space by moving beyond the macro level sociological analyses of nursing, such as those which take women's work and dirty work as organising theoretical frameworks. While an understanding of nursing as women's work is useful at a macro (structural) level it does not provide us with a mechanism to tap the everyday experiences of working nurses or what they take for granted about the ways in which it is possible to have privileged access to other people's bodies. The dirty work framework is also useful for understanding nursing because it too can provide a macro level perspective, but the dirty work construct does not really establish why some jobs are considered dirty and others not, given that dirtiness does not necessarily inhere in tasks designated as dirty.

Through the 'window' of nurses' work experiences of the body we can better understand the body in society, not only in the sense of how women's traditional roles have involved caring for others (which is central in nursing) but also how that is done when the work in question is designated as 'dirty' and when it is taboo and hidden from public view. This study, therefore, attempts to analyse things which feminists have identified as typically sex-typed female tasks, and roles which have been limited by an inadequate space in which to articulate them – in the sense that they are of low status, unrecognised, undervalued, privatised, invisible, and unproductive (in an economic Marxist sense). As well, it is a study of highly sophisticated and subtle social skills which nurses (mostly women) have developed to deal with what they know is potentially or actually embarrassing, threatening, frightening, and unfamiliar for patients. In essence it is a study of the privatised and professional everyday working lives of nurses, and hence it is about things which are not available to public scrutiny or to the average sociological researcher.

METHODOLOGICAL ISSUES

Macro level analyses provide us with abstractions of everyday life, but the knowledge nurses accumulate through the experiences of dealing interactively and intimately with people is not abstract knowledge – though it is possible to draw abstractions from it. When nurses deal with the bodies of other people they operate from a knowledge base which is interpretive, contextual, and integrative of object and subject – it is what I have called a *somological* approach. It is the sort of knowledge which comes from practical professional experience. I wanted to tap that professional knowledge in order to build an understanding of the body in society. This study was conducted, therefore, with five major methodological challenges:

(1) It was about taboo and hitherto largely invisible and unresearched topics;

(2) It was about the details of professional nursing practice which concern the intimate aspects of other people's bodies and lived experience during illness, recovery and dying, in which case it was a sensitive topic;

(3) It was a study conducted about a subject which had inherent epistemological and theoretical difficulties and for which there was no one single adequate methodological framework;

(4) The subject matter was familiar to me in the sense that I knew about these things in a way which had not yet been translated into language, that is, it was about the things I learned to take for granted as a nurse, and which I wanted to be made explicit; and

(5) I was researching the knowledge of nurses who were predominantly expert practitioners and who could not always easily describe what they know.

Each of these five factors had direct implications for the theoretical and methodological approach which the topic demanded. However, my background as a nurse allowed me access to the knowledge which nurses have, and in that sense one of these constraints could also be advantageous if I could use it in conjunction with established and appropriate methods of research.

Because nursing practice is heavily influenced by experience, the researcher must share the same professional experience in order to decide what questions to ask nurses, if indeed the researcher wishes to get at the very essence of nursing practice. This is a study which must be grounded in more than abstractions and observable reality because nurses may not deliberately think about their practice until someone like me asks them to explain why they do certain things – that is, to explain what they take for granted. Additionally, because I was researching silent, taboo, and hidden aspects of social life, the methodology would need to allow for that. One persistent feature of research involving nurses' work is the extent to which researchers have asked the 'wrong' questions (see Lublin 1984). There is also a general trend in research in the health care area which results in nurses being ignored, undervalued, or invisible. Oakley (1984:24) noted this when she 'confessed' (her term) that during a '15 year career as a sociologist studying medical services' she had 'been particularly blind to the contribution made by nurses to health care'.

My research was designed to explore very deliberately what nurses know and take for granted. As a consequence of my own professional background, my research questions were derived not only from the literature but also from my experience as a nurse and a researcher. I was interested in the generalised social methods which nurses use to manage the body. Some of these methods help to structure situations so that they become manageable for the patient, and for the nurse, at times when high levels of intimacy and trust are required. They are also designed to manage embarrassment. Without these methods nurses' work would be impossible.

Research questions

The research questions centred around one pivotal theme – what made nursing care socially possible, what were the major obstacles in transgressing normal social rules and what normal social rules,

are suspended, or alternatively, which context-specific rules apply
in nursing? In effect, I wanted to know how nurses construct a view
of the body which allows them to function as practitioners whose
role involves transgressing taken-for-granted rules governing normal
social relations and the body in 'civilised' society. I wanted to
explore the specific problems created by this rule-breaking (if indeed
it was rule-breaking) and the practices which are employed to
counter or manage such situations when rule-breaking concerns
the body. Specifically I wanted to know:

(1) How, in becoming nurses, they overcome what they have
been socialised to believe about the body, body exposure, and
body accessibility in our culture;

(2) What they remember of the first time they performed
body care for another;

(3) What occupationally-specific methods they learn which
facilitate doing their work, especially those aspects of it which
are invasive of the body, and which therefore give rise to
potential and actual embarrassment;

(4) How the context of care is constructed so that it is socially
permissible to touch the body to provide nursing care;

(5) How nurses negotiate the social territory of doing for
patients what they would normally do for themselves in private;

(6) How they manage when they must touch those parts of
body which are proscribed, and how they construct these
encounters with patients so that this level of intimacy is possible;

(7) How they manage sexuality and sexual behaviour during
body care, and what they do when the situation becomes
problematic;

(8) How they manage the body care of dying patients and the
dead body;

(9) How they care for others when the tasks to be performed
are potentially or actually nauseating, or truly awful;

(10) How they help people cope with a dysfunctional,
disfigured, deformed, or damaged body in illness experience;

(11) How they recognise embarrassment and manage it;

(12) How they purposefully and deliberately help patients
with situations that would generally be considered embarrassing;

(13) How patients make the nurse's job easier or more
difficult during body care, and what particular patient behaviours
facilitate or hamper the nurse's activities;

(14) How they manage an occupation which concerns aspects

of life normally kept from public view and not discussed openly, and which may be considered dirty or sexual;

(15) How they manage nursing care of the body when the patient has a high public profile or high status.

The questions I had posed would be difficult to answer, not only because they concerned delicate and sensitive subject matter, but also because they concerned the very basis of nursing practice — that is, the things which nurses seem to do routinely in the course of their everyday practice. The questions, therefore, appeared to be both very complex and, simultaneously, very simple, but they raised very difficult methodological problems. How is it possible, for example, to research things which are by nature hidden, and around which there is considerable silence? How is it possible to make explicit those things which nurses take for granted? How is it possible to start research in an area where what is known is not written down or explicitly articulated?

THEORETICAL CONSIDERATIONS

The specific theoretical backgrounds which informed the research approach to this study are drawn from grounded theory, ethnomethodology, and Garfinkel's (1967) notion of disrupted social order – a specific technique within the ethnomethodological framework. The particular research techniques employed to collect the data were chosen to take account of the methodological problems outlined above. I combined observation (of different types) and in-depth interviews, and the interviews were adapted to take account of the sensitivities of the topic.

The application of this particular combination of theoretical and research approaches takes account of the inadequacy of studying nursing only in a logico-positivist way, and of the need to document what has been unexplored. As a first measure it was necessary to study nurses in their 'natural' surroundings and to plot the major concepts and parameters of their daily work, and later, to ask them to explain (in so far as this is possible) what they do and why. In this sense, however, I had the added difficulty of the lack of theoretical space for the body – I could not study the body within any particular theoretical stance because the space for such work did not exist.

Grounded theory, therefore, offered great potential for my topic because it provides the framework for starting almost from a blank slate, so to speak. It allows the researcher to inductively build a theory about the social world by allowing the field to inform the course and theoretical outcome(s) of the research. It does not necessarily impose on the researcher any preconceived ideas about the eventual nature of any theory which might emerge from the work, though, I am sceptical about the notion that the researcher goes into the field without any preconceived ideas at all. Field and Morse (1985:Ch. 1) see great advantages in grounded theory for nursing. This is particularly so for those

who are attempting to identify unknown or unclear phenomenon [because] the current state of underlying theory development in relation to research questions of relevance to nurses require that more attention be paid to the development of concepts and the reality of the context in which they occur (Field & Morse 1985:6–7).

Grounded theory provided the scope to theorise areas of social life which have not so far been well studied, and where I had little to lead me, other than literature which told me the topics I wanted to explore were dealt with largely by silence and invisibility. One of the fundamental principles of grounded theory, as Glaser and Strauss (1967) described it, is that it allows theory to arise from data. It is a way of generating theory which is grounded in data taken from real and naturalistic settings. It is, in this way, a very pure kind of theory because it does not presuppose any particular perspective or way of looking at a problem. It was ideal for my purposes because I wanted to study nurses going about the ordinary everyday business of nursing care. While it was possible to follow the fundamental processes of grounded theory which Glaser and Strauss (1967) outlined (that is, by using theoretical sampling and comparisons from different sources, memo writing, and generating theory and verifying it), grounded theory alone would not allow me to focus my attention on how, exactly, nurses manage their work. Ethnomethodology, though, provides an approach which is not only philosophically compatible with grounded theory, but which also allows the researcher to concentrate on the ways in which people actively make their social lives manageable and meaningful. Not only that, it emphasises the particular social (interpersonal and intrapersonal) strategies (methods) which contribute to a meaningful construction of social life, and I was particularly interested in the strategies which nurses use.

The combination of ethnomethodology and grounded theory provides a solution to the difficulty of working on subject matter where little is known but where there is a simultaneously need to know **how** nurses manage the demands of body care in 'civilised' society. Grounded theory provides the framework for generating theory while ethnomethodology contributes the perspective whereby the researcher focuses on how people make sense of the world and what rules they assume underlie the taken-for-granted. In the context of nursing, normal social rules are somehow suspended in relation to body exposure, physical intimacy and touch. This is where Garfinkel's notion of disrupted social order is applicable. Sharrock and Anderson (1986:29–33) describe how Garfinkel became famous for devising 'experiments' where he and his students deliberately disrupted social order by breaking taken-for-granted rules, such as behaving inappropriately in familiar contexts. These experiments were designed to make social rules explicit as organising elements of social life in which one assumes a high level of mutual understanding about what it 'normal'. It is not considered 'normal', for example, for people to subject themselves to the sorts of practices which nurses engage in with patients – rather, nursing takes place in a specific context and it is constructed as such. Although it is common sense knowledge that nurses do certain intimate things, the particular details of their work is highly privatised and not necessarily widely known unless people have had personal experience of hospitalisation. Nurses are allowed privileged access to other people's bodies, but how is it possible for nurses and patients to relate to each other if there is a disruption of the normal social rules which apply in society generally? This was a fundamental question, which, if answered, had the potential to illustrate how the body is constructed and managed in social life. Even allowing for the occupationally specific latitude given to nurses in their professional role, an analysis of their work had the potential to yield valuable information about the body in 'civilised' society because nursing is practised in a particular cultural context; it is not a de-culturised activity.

Research design

The study was conducted in two major stages and it took place over a four year period. The first stage involved two kinds of observational data collection to identify and code the major concepts in the form of a working theory. This particular approach was adopted because, firstly, little was known about the subject matter of the study, and secondly, there was a need to observe the natural setting of nursing practice in order to start identifying fundamental practices and concepts. Field and Morse (1985:75) argue that in circumstances such as this, observation allows access to events which may not be explored in interviews because the interviewees may not think to tell the researcher – that is, they take them for granted.

This working theory and its component concepts formed the basis of the second stage, that is, in-depth interviews with 34 nurses. From these interviews I refined the working theory into a grounded theory of the management of the body in nursing — what I came to call *somology*. The interviews were constructed on the basis of the theoretical sampling (Glaser & Strauss 1967:Ch. 3) from the observational work. These interviews allowed me to talk with the people whose work I had been observing and to ask them to explain, in as much detail as they could, how their work with other people's bodies was managed as a social and professional process.

A qualitative approach, using both observation and interviews, and taking ethnomethodology and grounded theory as my philosophical and theoretical context, allowed me to make taken-for-granted aspects of nurses' work explicit and, in the case of the body where so much silence exists, to establish a dialogue between the researcher and the researched, which is essential. Such a dialogical approach is necessary because ample evidence exists (see Lublin 1984 for example) to illustrate that interactive methodologies are required for researching some aspects of nursing practice.

The combination of research methods I selected provided a way of maximising the validity and reliability of my theory. My observations and the concepts I derived from them were validated and refined repeatedly as the interviews proceeded, and I asked experienced nurses to tell me how and why they did things – the interviewees were a test of validity and reliability, because I had to present to them for verification the things which I had observed, and which I theorised were taken for granted in their everyday working lives. In doing this, I had to cause them to think through and put into words what they knew – a process which requires a high level of reciprocity (Schutz 1962).

The observational data, therefore, served to establish the baseline concepts, which were explored in detail and refined, particularly in respect of the rules which operate in nursing care of the body. They also formed part of a triad design consisting of observational data in which I was firstly a visitor and secondly a patient, and of interview data. There was, therefore, a triangulation of methods –

a process which enhances the validity and reliability of the study and which contributes to the ability to generalise from it.

THE OBSERVATIONAL DATA

As a 'native' (Schwartz & Jacobs 1979:48–49) of hospitals it is easy for me to gain access to the field and to become part of the local environment. As a known nurse and academic my presence in (some) hospitals is not unusual, although the purpose for my being in a particular place at a particular time usually requires explanation. In order, therefore, for me to do a block of field work for this study I needed a good cover because I did not want people to know I was 'making observations' or 'doing research'. I did not want anything unusual to appear to be happening while I focused my attention on this aspect of the study. The known observer can, by his or her presence, disturb the natural environment which causes a change in normal behaviour (Field & Morse 1985:79) and consequently the researcher can record unreliable data.

There was, however, an ethical issue to be considered if I was to do unobtrusive (covert or secretive) observational work. Some authors (for example, Field & Morse 1985:76) believe such measures are never defensible, however, others disagree. Lofland and Lofland (1984:21–24) argue that one needs to consider what they call 'open' and 'closed' settings, as well as whether or not the researcher is engaged in covert activities. They define 'open' settings as places where 'in law and tradition' any person 'has a right to be', such as airports and bus stops, whereas 'closed' settings are defined as those where not just 'anybody' can go and where the researcher needs to negotiate access (Lofland & Lofland 1984:21–22). In my case, my setting fell somewhere between the two – I was concerned with a relatively open place (a hospital) but where not everyone has a 'right' to be. That is, one is expected to have some specific purpose to be in a hospital, but in the Australian context, they are relatively public places.

The question of secrecy was clarified well by Roth when he observed that

All research is secret in some ways and to some degree – we never tell the subjects 'everything'. We can escape the secrecy more or less completely only by making the subjects participants in the research effort, and this process, if carried far enough, means there will be no more 'subjects'. So long as there exists a separation of the role between the researchers and those researched upon, the gathering of information

will inevitably have some hidden aspects even if one is an openly
declared observer (1970:278).

Roth (1970:279) also highlights that we are, as social scientists,
always engaged in the process of observation.

Most of us, in fact, never cease observing the social sphere about us and
are continually interpreting the behaviour of people about us. Some of
these observations are systematically organized into a 'research project',
but most of the observations and interpretations are casual and are
never recorded. But there are obviously all levels of observation and
interpretation between these extremes and the appropriate place for a
boundary line remains a moot point (Roth 1970:279).

I had been doing small pieces of observational field work as I went
about my normal work-related activities (such as doing some hospital-based work in relation to my normal teaching responsibili-
ties), but I also needed some time to be an observer without the
distractions which come from being a participant-as-observer (see
Field & Morse 1984:76–77). The ideal opportunity to do some
sustained field work arose when a close friend required relatively
major surgery and she was admitted to a small private hospital.
Both of us were known to many of the staff so my extended visits
over a five day period were not seen by them as unusual. I spent the
time not only doing the things one does when visiting friends in
hospital, but also making field notes and marking assignments. My
cover remained intact, although some staff wanted to know how I
could have a job which allowed me, seemingly, never to work. To
these people I replied that I had brought a batch of assignments
and that I could mark them anywhere.

While I was well aware of the ethical considerations inherent in
using this situation for collecting data, I was also legitimately in the
field as a visitor, and it was inevitable that I would find this time
rich in ideas and data, and that it would contribute to my thinking
on the ways in which nurses manage other people's bodies. I took
advantage, opportunisticly, of a naturally occurring event. Lofland
and Lofland (1984:23) take the view that

there are very serious, perhaps damning, ethical problems in *all* covert
research if the presumed immorality of deception is the overriding
concern. Deception is no less present in public and open setting
research than in preplanned, 'deep cover' research in closed settings.
On the other hand, if other concerns are also important (for example,
lack of harm to those researched, or the theoretical importance of a
setting which can never be studied openly), then we can find no more
justification for abolishing *all* deep cover research, preplanned or not,
than for abolishing secret research in public settings.

Because the opportunity to do some valuable field work had presented itself, I was particularly observant and made notes on things which I needed to explore more thoroughly. My primary role, however, remained that of visitor and friend to the person I was visiting, and my status as researcher was secondary. In this situation I could be both a friend and visitor, and simultaneously, I could be a researcher because my reflections on the way people behaved toward me (as a visitor) were the very stuff of my research project. It was naturalistic research in real and uncontrived circumstances. Before I progressed to any further data collection, however, I talked with the Director of Nursing of the hospital and told her about my note taking. This did not surprise her because I was known as an avid people watcher anyway, and I was simply being my 'normal' self.

As a visitor, I was able to observe the daily activity from the viewpoint of a researcher and ethnographer. During this time I was able to identify and develop many of the ideas which formed my working theory and which I later explored in the interviews. For example, I knew that nurses preferred to do much of their work without relatives and visitors present and that they usually asked them to leave the room when they tended to the patient. This practice also extended to me, a known nurse, but also a visitor, and, to the staff, my status as visitor was dominant in this context. On several occasions I was asked to leave while various care procedures were conducted. There were some exceptions to this when I was very well known to the attending nurse and had an established relationship extending over many years, but even then some staff were not comfortable about my presence, and I waited outside the room during various nursing activities. I was able to explore this more fully in the interviews which followed.

This period also enabled me to identify what appeared to be a taken-for-granted trajectory toward recovery, and I identified the signals which nurses took to mean that a patient was, or was not, progressing at the perceived 'normal' rate. This trajectory was accompanied by a re-negotiation of how dependent the patient was on the nurse for assistance with body care. As the patient regained independence, nurses invaded less and less of the patient's body space, inquired less about a range of body functions, and the level of surveillance was progressively reduced. During this time I also noted that both language and the manner of discourse about body products and body functions were problematic. Not only was there a need to talk to patients about things which patients would not normally discuss, such as bowel movements, but this was also an ever-present difficulty for all parties and it required particular management. As a nurse I am familiar with the problem because of my own experiences, but I was interested to locate the problems of language and discourse in a more interpretive and integrative social framework. I was able to observe that 'civilised' body functions required a style of discourse which ensured at least partial privacy, and later I explored this more fully in the interviews. These five days of observation, which covered the period of admission to discharge of the person I was visiting, contributed to the scope and content of the interviews which followed. Several months later I had another opportunistic occasion for some field work when I was admitted to hospital for elective surgery. Although this event was unrelated to my research project, it was inevitable that my experience would contribute to my research, as had been the case of other sociological researchers who found themselves admitted to hospital and discovered the temptation for recording their experiences was irresistible (see Fairhurst 1977, Hyndman 1985). I took the opportunity to reflect purposefully on my own experiences (as a patient this time rather than a nurse or visitor/friend), to make field notes and, when the opportunity arose, to talk informally to some of the staff about aspects of nursing practice. Strauss (1987:11) says that such experiential data 'not only give added theoretical sensitivity but provide a wealth of provisional suggestions for making comparisons, finding variations, and sampling widely on theoretical grounds'. They contribute also to the formulation of 'conceptually dense and carefully ordered theory' (Strauss 1987:11).

However, in contrast to others who have studied the experience of patienthood through their own experience (Fairhurst 1977, Hyndman 1985), I am, as a (sometimes) practising nurse, very familiar with routines in hospital life. I was able to concentrate more on the social aspects of these routines and on my own reactions and feelings.

I was hospitalised for ten days, during which time I required little assistance with anything after the first two days, so I had plenty of time for observation and reflection on my own experiences. During this time it became apparent to me that the nature of the nurse-patient relationship and 'the manner' of the nurse were central to the management of the body and its various functions, embarrassment, and the patient's sense of vulnerability. I was also able to further develop the concept of the recovery trajectory. I later explored each of these observations in the interviews.

THE INTERVIEWS

A semi-structured interview schedule (developed from the observation data and from the literature) was trialed with two colleagues (both academic nurses), one male and one female, both of whom are familiar with the methodology I was using. No major changes seemed necessary so I proceeded to interview an additional 32 nurses. I was later to discover, however, that because of what was being revealed in the interviews, my schedule had not addressed the issues of sexuality and its relationship to nursing as explicitly as some of the interviewees indicated it should have. These constant comparisons (Glaser & Strauss 1967) contributed substantially to the refinement of my theory of somology and produced minor modifications to the interview so that sexuality became more centrally tied to the notion of embodied existence and body management in nursing. I was aware when interviewing of the difficulties Oakley (1981) encountered when she studied the experience of childbirth, because, in her case, the textbooks had provided little guidance for the immediate and practical difficulties she faced when her interviewees looked to her for support and information during labour. I expected that many of my interviewees might not be comfortable with the subject matter I wanted to discuss, particularly issues related to sexuality and sexual expression, which was one topic area which caused me to deviate from textbook models of interviewing.

At the time of commencing this work I was not aware of any literature other than Oakley's (1981) work that helped the researcher interview people on sensitive and taboo topics. I sometimes found myself in situations where I knew I was talking about things which are highly sensitive and often regarded as very private matters. At these times I was delving into subject matter akin to incest and rape, because I was asking about things which make women feel vulnerable, exploited, and sometimes guilty. As a researcher one does not go into such matters without considering the potentially traumatising (or therapeutic) effects of discussing such issues. I had to be very careful how I asked certain questions. For example, if I asked 'have you ever been sexually harassed by a patient?' the answer was usually 'no'. But if I asked if they had experienced situations where patients had made sexually explicit and uninvited advances toward them, or touched them in intimate ways, the answer was often 'yes' and they related instances about particular patients. I was later to discover that Cowles (1988) had experienced similar difficulties; she had called these 'sensitive topics' and they required the researcher to take a much more empathic and supportive role than is usually suggested as appropriate.

Language selection was also difficult at times, and, while the texts often stress the need to use language familiar to the interviewee, and they emphasise the importance of phrasing the questions to fit the interviewee's frame of reference, there is little to help the researcher to talk about some of the things that were relevant to my study. I occasionally found myself relying more on my training and experience as a nurse than on my training and experience as a social researcher, though the two share many common elements.

In deviating from the (recommended) detached stance of the researcher, I became involved in discussions about topics which carry a sometimes heavy emotional burden, and which are issues for us as nurses. It is not possible in such circumstances to retain the role of the researcher all the time, rather, it follows that in such encounters people talk as fellow members of the same professional group. In my study, that was a necessary component of the research process, and it is not possible to talk only in the roles of researcher and 'researchee'.

Later, when it came time to report my data analysis, I also took notice of Cowles' (1988) comments on the methodological difficulties of studying sensitive topics, in her case the surviving friends and relatives of murder victims. She described how the textbook does not always help researchers who are dealing with emotionally charged and sensitive issues. Though Cowles' (1988) work was not published until after I had collected my data, it confirmed my experience that what has been written in textbooks on interviewing techniques has, in the main, excluded the sorts of situations and issues in which I was interested. That is, they have avoided discussing the emotions which often accompany research of this kind, and they have generally not been helpful for the researcher who is exploring topics which people normally do not discuss. In some interviews, therefore, I sometimes had to lead and probe and look for non-verbal signs, rather than rely only on verbal interaction. The discomfort that was sometimes apparent when I asked about some topics supported my view that the body is a problem in our culture, and that researching its management in nursing is a sometimes delicate matter.

I was also later to read Cannon's (1989) report of the 'emotional pain' of interviewing people about stressful and sensitive topics. In her case, she was concerned with women undergoing treatment for breast cancer – a process she described as requiring compromise and negotiation because the textbook models of qualitative methodology did not allow for what she encountered. She explains how she quite specifically made an emotional input into her encounters with the women she interviewed in order to establish the trust she needed to find out what it felt like to have cancer of the breast. While my study did not involve the level of emotionality one would suppose Cannon (1989) experienced, I was, nevertheless, asking about highly sensitive and emotional matters – the sort of things people often do not want to tell anyone.

To adapt the interviews specifically to suit my subject matter, I asked questions about areas of practice where I suspected the interface between professional culture and 'normal' social culture would be in conflict. For example, if nurses had to care for people they knew socially, would this represent a disruption of social order as Garfinkel's experiments had (Sharrock & Anderson 1986:Ch. 3)? When they first started their professional careers, it would be reasonable to expect that they would transgress what they had learned about the underlying rules about the body in society. I wanted to problematise these times in order to identify the social rules — a process which Garfinkel had used successfully.

Another adaptation I used was to tell the interviewees about what I had observed in my field work and ask them if they could tell me about the reasons for various practices, such as sending the relatives and visitors away. I also outlined a small scenario (which I later came to call *minifisms*) to explore one very specific way in which nurses make the body manageable. Having outlined the scenario, I asked the interviewees if they could tell me why nurses did such things and what functions they had. Their responses (and the scenario) are discussed in detail in Chapter 7.

The interviewees

The sample of 34 interviewees consisted of 27 registered nurses (2 of whom were retired), 2 students in their third (and final) year of a pre-registration diploma program, and 5 enrolled nurses. There were 4 males and 30 females, making the male/female proportions approximate to those in the Australian nursing workforce generally. They ranged in age from 19 years to over 60 years (the precise age was not revealed), with the largest number (N=13) being in their 30s, and about equal numbers in their 20s (N=8) and 40s (N=7).

They were all either engaged in, or had previously been engaged in clinical roles.

The interviewees have a wide range of experience, which covers all areas of specialisation in nursing, but because I was predominantly interested in the adult body, the sample does not include many with extensive experience in children's nursing, although there are several who have worked in this field. The sample was chosen so that all areas of specialisation were covered, and in favour of those with at least 5 years experience of clinical practice. The 2 participants who had less than 5 years experience were students. They were included in order that all current groups in nursing could be sampled. (The mean number of years of experience = 14.33, s.d. = 8.41 years.)

The reasons for sampling from more experienced nurses were: firstly, I believed that they would be more comfortable with the socially sensitive areas of their work; and secondly, I wanted to sample as many expert practitioners as possible (see Benner 1982a, 1984, Benner & Tanner 1987, Benner & Wrubel 1988) because they would be more likely to articulate the more subtle aspects of practice, and I was interested in what they had learned from experience. It is a reasonable cross section of the nursing workforce, although skewed in favour of more experienced nurses.

As a group, they were a well qualified sample of nurses,[2] with thirteen of them having tertiary education. With respect to the nursing qualifications of the registered nurses[3] all were registered to practise general nursing, 12 were also registered midwives, 5 held qualifications in the acute care/intensive care/coronary care area, and 2 were registered to practise psychiatric nursing. In addition, 3 held certificates in mothercraft, 1 in ophthalmic nursing and 1 in orthopaedics.

They revealed a strong bias toward British ancestry with English being the most common in this sample. The ethnic backgrounds of those I interviewed had some influence on their early experiences as nurses because of the way they were socialised at home (discussed in Chapter 5).

THE DATA: HOW DO NURSES MANAGE THE BODY?

In keeping with the grounded theory process I had adopted for this project, data analysis began very early in the study with memo writing and preliminary and provisional theory building during the periods of field observations (Strauss 1987:Ch. 5, Glaser & Strauss 1967) and it continued. In grounded theory, data analysis is an ongoing process – it is inductive and therefore the theory is never completed, rather, one gets closer to an accurate theory the more data are analysed and verified.

When it came to analysing the data, I became aware that they did not fit models of knowledge that I had been taught to see as a social scientist. Nonetheless, the data 'felt' familiar to me as a nurse. I became aware that what I had researched was not knowledge which nurses had 'received' as some 'objective' reality, but knowledge derived from and accumulated through personal experience and practice. It was not immediately easy to describe in discrete thematic ways.

It became apparent from the data that sexuality was a major problem, particularly male sexuality, and that this was intimately connected to the way maleness and masculinity are constructed. I had made several memos early in the project about the need for sexual matters to have a prime place in my theory, and, throughout the collection and analysis of the interviews, sexuality increasingly emerged as a difficult area for nurses. Consequently, it has been incorporated here as a central consideration for a theory of the body in nursing.

Each of the other major themes in the data has been taken as the organisational basis for the chapters which form Part II of this book, and they illustrate how the body is fundamentally and essentially a genderised and sexualised construct around which many aspects of social life are organised. So important is sexuality/body in our culture and so central is it to nurses' work that it recurs as a theme throughout the following chapters.

The theory of somology which is described here is an attempt to draw some more general conclusions about the body, in particular, how it features within a theoretical construct about the work of nurses. In this way, the theory can transcend the data.

The book is in two parts. Part I is a critique of the nursing and social science literature on the body. Chapter 1 examines the literature on the body in nursing theory and practice. Chapter 2 examines the ways in which the body has been conceptualised and theorised, particularly in philosophy, history and sociology. Chapter 3 discusses aspects of social life in which the body has been explicitly studied in relation to what Norbert Elias' (1978) called the 'civilising process', and in anthropology and psychology. Chapter 4 analyses the intimate relationship between the body and sexuality. These four chapters are crucial to understanding the research data because they not only provide the essential background for understanding the nature of what was studied, but they also establish an awareness of the complexities of the body in social life and the sensitive nature of the issues that are explored in the chapters which form Part II. These early chapters, therefore, formally state the context in which the data are to be understood, and they provide a rationale which attempts to illustrate why empiricism and reduction will not lead to an adequate understanding of the body in social life. Chapters 5 to 10 analyse the empirical work for this study. Chapter 5 is a general introduction to what nurses learn about the social management of the bodies of others, how that learning compares with their socialised patterns of relating to others, especially as it concerns emotional control and language. Chapter 6 details specific methods which nurses learn as part of their occupational socialisation and professional practice and which make their work socially accept-able in the context of hospitalisation, and it deals with the structural and organisational aspects of that sociology of body. Chapter 7 analyses the more interpersonal and existential aspects of the practices which Chapter 6 describes. It also illustrates, in more detail, the somological approach to the body which nurses use. Chapter 8 deals specifically with the temporal dimensions of who controls the body during its 'handing over' from patient to nurse in illness and dying, and its 'handing back' from nurse to patient in recovery. Chapter 9 is concerned with sexuality in nursing and the problem of the sexualised body. Although sexuality is a feature of discussions in other sections of this study, Chapter 9 examines this issue in its own right as a central problematic of the body for nurses. Chapter 10 shifts the emphasis from 'the problem of the body' within nurses' work, to the wider social and public consequences of that work because of the underlying 'problem of the body'. As is the practice with material of this kind, the data are reported verbatim from transcripts of the interviews. I resisted the temptation to sanitise or launder some of the language and I expect some people may find parts of it offensive in this 'civilised' society of ours. I decided there was no point in continuing to hide the body and its management from public view, especially in a study where I am attempting to make that aspect of social life more explicit. Furthermore, the language which the interviewees use is often so graphic that any attempt on my part to 'clean it up' would detract from its impact.

From my own viewpoint, I had to overcome a sense of (learned) inhibition in order to report some of the material. In particular the data which deal with very basic aspects of human existence, such as excreta, are not regarded as appropriate topics of conversation in most social settings. Throughout the course of this research, when I have been asked what I am studying, I have become acutely aware of the need to choose my words carefully when I describe what I am doing. For instance, if I said I was researching a sociology of the body, people did not know what that meant. If I said that I was interested in how nurses managed other people's bodies and body products, I often perceived that some people (non-nurses) were reluctant to pursue the conversation any further. Some, however, were intrigued by what I was doing and expressed great interest in the project. I am aware, though, that I have been researching a taboo topic and that there are possible negative consequences of that for me (see Faberow 1963). For example, there have been instances over the last five years when people have indicated to me that the things I was researching were best ignored and kept private.

The following chapters attempt to explain these reactions in relation to 'the problem of the body'. Nurses, whose work involves them so intimately with the body, are also members of society, and they are not immune from the beliefs and norms which influence social behaviour.

Postscript to the study

There are several interesting events which occurred in the aftermath of this research. Some of these events were deliberately constructed by me in order to test reaction to my analyses and some events were spontaneous. I modified some of my concepts and terminology in response to comments made by two of the interviewees, who read an advanced draft of the data analysis. I have talked to others, both formally and informally about what I was researching. What is reported here is, in part, a reflection of their reactions as well as my analysis of what the data mean to me.

In response to people's reactions I revised the chapters which concerned the notion of somological practice because while the two interviewees knew well what was intended in this concept and they liked the term, they argued that the way I had described it then, was perhaps too subtle for anyone other than a nurse to understand, and that this was because of the very reason I was arguing – that it is not received and objective knowledge. I also used the word 'privatised' in place of Elias' (1978) term, 'civilised', to more accurately reflect the way in which the body is dealt with in social life. The notion of 'civilisation' is not as descriptive as 'privatisation' and the latter is more applicable in nursing contexts.

The issue of sexuality (and its relation to sensuality) is by far the most interesting and intriguing aspect of this research, and I have but scraped the surface. I recognise now, with the benefit of hindsight and experience, that the sample does not adequately represent the views of men in nursing, and that this is a function of the extent to which the male body is fundamental to notions of maleness and masculine power, and to patriarchy. It would therefore be useful for a similar study to be conducted by a male researcher with male nurses. There is also an unexplained atmosphere of fear about the sexualised body, and there are some ways in which we view the body which can only be described as mysterious and superstitious. This is true not only of women in their dealings with men, but it is also probably true for men (according to one person – a male) because men react to the power of women's reproduction, the mysterious and hidden organs of reproduction, and most of all, the hormones!

There is a mystery about the body and the power of sexuality which this study has hinted at and which is worthy of further investigation. It is similar in many ways to the mystery and fear which surrounds death – an attitude which would seem to have some of the characteristics that might be expected in a non-industrialised and non-scientised culture. My analysis of this material has left me with the firm impression that, with respect to the dead body, we are culturally very superstitious and fearful, or, at the very least, discomforted. I do not know why that is so, nor do my data give any indication of likely reasons beyond the possibility that our dominant world view promotes science as the most powerful way of knowing, yet science is deficient when it comes to knowing about death. And while science has illuminated some aspects of embodied sexuality, it has almost entirely focused on objective reality and not existential reality (personal meaning, physical experience, sensuality and the like).

There are a number of recurrent themes in this research. First, there is the extent to which men have power over women, how this is often expressed bodily, and how male and female bodies are conceptualised differently. As one person remarked, 'male bodies are seen in terms of power, the female body in terms of its problems. The only good thing about the female body [in the perceptions of men] is if it's worth looking at or fucking.' Another recurrent theme is the extent to which nursing knowledge and nursing practice do not fit comfortably into positivist scientific frameworks and will not do so until there is a paradigm shift. Such a shift may come with changing societal attitudes to such things as the value of work that women and nurses do. A third theme is the invisibility of nurses' work and the relationship of this to women's work in general, and to the privatised body in particular. Again it is recognised that such invisibility is likely to continue until such time as there is a shift in our cultural definitions of acceptable public behaviour with respect to the body.

A fourth theme which recurs is the problem of language, not only in reference to privatised bodily functions, but also with the inability to articulate what nurses do when they practise. The analyses of the term, 'doing nothing' is seen as a particularly vivid illustration of this problem.

A fifth theme, and one which is potentially controversial in nursing, is the notion that somological practice is not necessarily holistic. For me to argue that nurses, especially experienced and expert practitioners like those interviewed for this study, do not practise holisticly is to attack an ideological cornerstone in nursing. These data, as I analyse and interpret them, do not support the idea that nurses practise holisticly (meaning that they consider **all** aspects of a person – social, biological, medical, pathological, spiritual, psychological, and so on). The data, however, do support the idea that expert nurses acknowledge the embodied existence of their patients, that they take account of the person as well as the body, and that they integrate various aspects of patients' and nurses' experiences of giving care into a composite and integrative view. They consider what is relevant and they make judgements about what is relevant based on the context of the particular circumstances (patients and situations) with which they are concerned. To me, this is something quite different from caring for 'the whole person' (whatever that means) in a way which encourages surveillance and a comprehensive survey of the patient's nursing (read social and life) history.

In addition to the follow-up interviews, I have talked to groups of students in pre-registration and post-registration nursing programs at the university where I work. I have outlined my data about embarrassment, the management of nakedness and intimate body care, and dying and recovery and its relationship to the ways the body is managed, and I have talked about sexuality in nursing practice. Without exception such sessions have been followed by requests from students that we concentrate more on these topics. The students want to learn more about the social management of the body. Clearly there are educational implications in this work for nurses.

During some of these teaching sessions I have been told by some of the young male students that sexual harassment is not just a problem for their female colleagues, that female patients sometimes 'accidentally' touch the nurse's genitalia during body care; that this is not uncommon, but men tend to laugh about it. It is not taken seriously by the men although they may be surprised by it when it happens. It seems that female advances where body contact is initiated by women provoke from men an altogether different reaction from the case when men touch women. This is a topic for further research and one which is beyond the scope of my data.

I have also had many opportunities to talk informally to non-nurses about what I have been researching, and almost without exception people have wanted to talk about their experiences of hospitalisation. This has been a rich and fascinating experience for me because men have talked (and seemed to have a 'need' to talk) of their sensual and sexual confusion during body care episodes which felt nice and comforting, but which they also found pleasantly arousing – an arousal which they felt to be socially inappropriate. They talked of not knowing how to behave toward a nurse, particularly one who was young and warm and attractive, and who did such sensual things to a man's body as wash and massage his back.

Like any research, this study has raised many questions and it has identified many areas for further work. One of the most obvious is the need to talk with patients about similar things to those I discussed with nurses, and I have started to explore this area; there is a need to talk more about these things with nurses who are male; there is an obvious area for further research in the areas of sexuality and its relationship to embodiment; and there is a need to explore so called 'basic' nursing care, that is, body care, more thoroughly. For example, how does it feel, existentially, to be dependent on, and to be handled by, others? One of the most neglected and potentially valuable areas for further work is in the area of how nurses view their own bodies, their illnesses, their experiences as patients themselves, and their need to sometimes be dependent on others. My own experience as a patient, which is reported in Chapter 7, caused me to comment not on how my medical care would be managed, but how I would be nursed and how I would respond to that care. Though I have not reported it here, some of my interview material contains comment on nurses as patients – they represent one of the most problematic groups to nurse. A number of intriguing questions could be explored. Why, for example, do nurses generally make either the very best or the very worst patients? Why do they sometimes neglect their own bodies and delay, often dangerously, seeking attention when they are ill? Why are they sometimes so stoic as patients and why are they sometimes the opposite? Why do they worry about whether or not they will be 'good' patients? What worries them about their own experiences of patienthood and why and how do their own experiences influence the way they practice?

NOTES

1. Empiricism is taken to mean an approach to the development of knowledge which: (1) relies fundamentally on human experience; (2) is able to be communicated in language – a necessary condition for the dissemination of ideas; (3) is usually, but not always derived from some form of deliberative research which is typically experimental in design; and (4) has come to share a relationship with positivism such that empiricism is assumed, in dominant ideologies of scientific knowledge, to require positivism. As a consequence, empiricism tends to produce knowledge which is reductive but which can be readily shared because it concerns those things for which there is some objective reality. Empirical research, as I define it and use the term here, is taken to mean the range of ways and methods by which it is possible to know and construct 'reality' (however it is defined by individuals) because all forms of experience contribute to perceiving and constructing reality. Although certain physiological capabilities are a necessary condition for empirically knowing the world, what one comes to regard as knowledge is a function of interaction between the biological and social.

2. The 1986 Australian census shows that of those qualified in nursing 0.46% also hold an award at the level of bachelor, and 1.89% at the level of diploma. (Source: Australian Institute of Health, Health Workforce Information Bulletin No. 13. Nurse Workforce 1986. Canberra, Australian Government Publishing Service.)

3. It is important when dealing with samples of registered nurses to take account of the area in which they practise. In Australia there have been several categories in which it was possible to register as a nurse (general, psychiatric, mental retardation, midwifery, geriatrics, mothercraft) and additional specialty areas, such as intensive care, where it is possible to hold additional qualifications. While there is variation in emphases in what (precisely) is practised among and within specialisations, there is also considerable commonality among areas of practice.

The Problem of the Body

1. The body and nursing

The occupation of nursing is fundamentally and centrally concerned with the care of other people's bodies, but it is care provided in a particular context. Physical body care and comfort are provided for those who are completely dependent on other people – the unconscious, the senile, the paralysed. But varying degrees of body care are required for most patients, according to their particular state of dependence. Nurses also help people with the experience of living with and through what is happening to their bodies during illness, recovery or dying – times when the body can dominate existence. Nurses are, therefore, centrally concerned with the object body (an objective and material thing) and the lived body (the body as it is experienced by living people). They are concerned with integrating the object body with the lived body. This is what I have termed *somology*, that is, understanding the body as an integration of the object body (the thing) into experience so that it is simultaneously an object, a means of experience, a means of expression, a manner of presence among other people, and a part of one's personal identity.

Benner and Wrubel (1988:82–89) indicate that nurses can help patients deal with the experience of illness as a process where lived and object body cannot be easily separated. My study reports data which illustrate how nurses manage the bodies of others, not only as objects – as they sometimes need to do to protect themselves and the patient from what is physically repulsive – but also how they do that in a way which does not disembody or objectify the person (patient). It is a study about expert nurses (see Benner 1982a, 1984), and to that extent it does not necessarily reflect the practice of nurses generally, because expert nurses provide examples of how nursing can be practised at best.

In recent decades, health care has been increasingly scientised and technologised and consequently there has been a tendency to de-emphasise those aspects of nursing which concern the physical care and comfort of patients – the nurturing aspects of nurses' work, although nurses have retained an ideological commitment to it. In nursing curricula, education, research and literature, there has been growing emphasis on the need for nurses to expand, develop and scientise their knowledge base and to theorise their practice.

However, what remains unchanged and unchanging is that nurses are fundamentally concerned with the physical care and comfort of patients – subject matter which does not readily lend itself to scientising, at least to the extent that science means objectification and reduction.

Nursing involves not only doing things which are traditionally assigned to females, and learning to do them by experience and practice, but also crossing social boundaries, breaking taboos and doing things for people which they would normally do for themselves in private if they were able. Berry (1986) has claimed, however, that nurses have not been taught how to manage crossing those boundaries. The data from this study overwhelmingly support her assertion, and they also show that body care, as nurses perform it, does not comfortably fit into a logic-positivist framework typical of mainstream science.

This chapter examines how nurses have written about the body in their work – theoretically, educationally, and socially, and it also describes how nurses have attempted to theorise and scientise their practice. It also traces ways in which the occupation of nursing has been analysed sociologically.

BODY CARE AND NURSES WORK

Nurses' work is not easily understood, nor is it easy to research because, as Melia (1979:58) has noted, 'nursing is a complex activity which is difficult to describe or define'. Additionally, our language is deficient in the area of women's reality generally, many aspects of nurses' work and nurses' knowledge are not accessible to positivist enquiry (Lublin 1984), and the body has been 'civilised' (Elias 1978), that is, it has become a private matter. Like other areas of women's work, nursing practice which concerns body care has been relatively neglected.

Goddard (1953 cited by Melia 1979:61) categorised (reduced) nurses' work into 'basic nursing' and 'technical nursing'. So-called 'basic nursing' originates from the physical needs of patients, and, irrespective of what ails patients, it is a universal characteristic of nursing. 'Technical nursing', on the other hand, is determined as a consequence of both the disease from which the patient suffers and medical interventions. Melia, however, is critical of these categories for two reasons. Firstly, Goddard's categorisation did not recognise the extent to which 'basic nursing' and 'technical nursing' interrelate for particular patients and depend on context (see also Benner 1982a, 1982b, 1984, Benner & Wrubel 1982, Benner & Tanner 1987, Munhall 1982a), and secondly, such categorisation denigrates those aspects of nursing care which are concerned with providing physical care and comfort – basic body care. She goes on to argue that

'Basic nursing' as a term has fallen into disrepute because it can be seen to imply lack of skill or importance. With the increase of intensive care and specialist units the term 'technical nursing' has gained momentum and prestige in recent years. There has been a tendency within the nursing profession to confuse the concept of a hierarchy of nursing skills with the notion of basic and technical nursing (Melia 1979:62).

McFarlane (1976) argues that the division of nursing care into 'basic' and 'technical' implies that the latter is more difficult than the former. So-called 'basic' care is truly basic, but basic in the sense that it is fundamental to the nursing care for any patient, and nurses use the term 'basic' to mean that such care is essential and concerned with first principles – the basis on which other things are established.

Traditionally, the work of nurses was organised into a hierarchy of tasks structured so that with increasing seniority one progressed from tasks of low status to those of higher status – a progression which not only reflected contemporary (scientific) management practices, but which also meant a move from more 'dirty' jobs to cleaner tasks usually associated with less contact with the bodies of other people – at least in the sense that one had to touch other people's bodies. Such an arrangement reflected qualities of relative cleanness or dirtiness, as well as status and seniority, and ascribed them to various tasks. In that system, body care and closely associated tasks, which were more likely to be dirty, had the lowest status. Body care was undertaken by nurses of the lowest professional status and least education, and this was believed to be appropriate. To some people, it is still appropriate. For example, during the much publicised time when the public hospital system in Australia could not attract enough registered nurses to maintain existing services, a spokesperson for the Royal College of Surgeons was quoted in a prominent Sydney newspaper as saying a solution lay in recruiting '[the] many young women . . . who could not find work'. Such people, he said, 'were willing to do the menial nursing tasks such as washing patients' (O'Neill 1987).

Nurses have maintained a paradoxical approach to 'basic' nursing care by assigning it low status with respect to who should perform it, yet simultaneously regarding it as profoundly important to the well-being and recovery of the patient. Nurses are ambivalent about body care – it is important and essential, but there is the question of who should perform it. In recent years, especially since the 1970s, there has been a move toward a more 'holistic' approach to the division of labour, so that the care of individual patients is provided on any one day (or shift) by the same nurse. More 'holistic' care means a shift in the division of labour toward an emphasis on the patient as an individual and away from an emphasis on the task to be performed. Consequently body care is no longer assigned to nursing staff of lowest status, however, there has been a trend to assign patients who have the lowest status value in terms of what could be called 'nursing care value' to staff of lowest status.

During the last several decades, and particularly since the 1950s, nurses have attempted to theorise their practice to bring the ideology and reality closer together, not only to give nursing greater legitimacy as a discipline, but also to use the products of their theorising in education.

THEORISING THE BODY IN NURSING

Historically, only a few nursing authors have attempted to address the problem of body care in nursing, and there has been a tendency to use language which camouflages or sanitises the body and some of its functions, while other authors have ignored the subject. Consequently the body has been absent or invisible, or it has had a vague presence. Nightingale, for instance, who was influential in many sanitary reforms in both public and private life in the nineteenth century, does not mention the body, or body care, as such, in her most famous text, *Notes on Nursing* (1969, first published in 1859). She refers to the body by inference in her chapter on 'Personal Cleanliness' in a way which focuses attention on the skin and the need to wash it thoroughly. She says:

The amount of relief and comfort experienced by sick after the skin has been carefully washed and dried, is one of the commonest observations made at a sick bed. But it must not be forgotten that the comfort and relief so obtained are not all. They are, in fact, nothing more than a sign that the vital powers have been relieved by removing something that was oppressing them. The nurse, therefore, must never put off attending to the personal cleanliness of her patient under the plea that all that is to be gained is a little relief, which can be quite as well given later (Nightingale 1969: Ch. XI).

A later nursing author to address the body was Virginia Henderson (1964). Even so, she locates body care as a very general or taken-for-granted and apparently self evident aspect of nursing. For Henderson, the body is implicit – a given.

The unique function of the nurse is to assist the individual, sick or well, in the performance of those activities contributing to health or its recovery (or to a peaceful death) that he [sic] would perform unaided if he had the necessary strength, will or knowledge. And to do this in such a way as to help him gain independence as rapidly as possible. This aspect of her [sic] work, this part of her function, she initiates and controls; of this she is master. In addition she helps the patient to carry out the therapeutic plan as initiated by the physician. She also, as a member of of a medical team, helps other members as they in turn help her, to plan and carry out the total program whether it be for the improvement of health, or the recovery from illness or support in death (Henderson 1964:8).

More recently Orem's (1980) theoretical stance continues in the directions taken by Henderson, but in Orem's work, the functions of nurses and the nature of nursing are expressed in terms of 'self care deficits' of patients. This approach is close to that taken by Henderson, yet in some ways it makes the body as an entity disappear. It is fragmented (reduced) into a range of self care deficits – in plain language these are aspects of physical care one cannot 'do for oneself', but which are part of normal daily life.

  The works of Nightingale, Henderson, and Orem are those in which there is an attempt to articulate the body in nursing care, but the body is either objectified and reduced or it is implicit. Henderson's definition of the functions of nurses, and Orem's model, although they have provided bases from which to empiri-cally investigate a range of nursing phenomena, including body care, are characterised by a coyness about the body and body care. The lack of space for the body in their writings may reflect attempts to fit it (and body care) into what they perceived to be the way(s) knowledge is constructed. Both of these writers theorised from their own experiences as nurses, but their work also shows how descriptions of nursing practice constructed within dominant para-digms of knowledge make nursing appear to be very simple and ordinary – it can have an appearance which is an artifact of the way it is described. However, that can also be a function of an impoverished language in relation to female reality (see, for example, Miller & Swift 1976, Spender 1985), and because nursing is an extension of traditional female roles it also suffers for want of an adequate discourse.

Parker (1988) argues for a more interpretive and phenomenological approach within which to theorise nursing. She gives an account of the patterns that have emerged over the last few decades from nursing's attempts to find a more appropriate (and independent) theoretical space in which to structure a very complex and difficult discipline like nursing. The medical model, while it deals overtly with the body, does so in a way which is reductionist and deterministic, and it stresses relationships of cause and effect. It is a model which is fundamentally mechanistic.

Nursing practice, however, is more interactive, more social, and more holistic. One cannot simply nurse the body in the bed. One must do business with it as a person because nursing means being able to view the body and the person as inseparable. Parker (1988:10) is one of a small number of nurses (see also Gadow 1980, 1982, Colliere 1986, Wolf 1986a, 1986b) who are beginning to develop a literature on the body because, as she says, 'as nurses we are witnesses again and again to the human struggle to transcend the boundedness of embodiment'. She summarised her position in these terms:

I wanted to reject what I saw as the overly rational reductionist medical model with its emphasis on diagnosis of pathophysiology and treatment of disease . . . [and] . . . I believed also that there was a need to conceptualise body in other than the reductionist biologistic understanding of the medical model . . . . I wanted to be able to capture the idea of body as lived experience, as subject rather than simply as the object of other people's inspection (Parker 1988:5).

The lived body, as Parker and others (Gadow 1980, 1982, Colliere 1986) discuss it, is relatively unresearched within nursing, but that is probably due in part to a trend in nursing toward scientising practice to be consistent with other disciplines.

SCIENTISING NURSING PRACTICE

There has been continuous debate about whether nursing is an art or a science. It has been variously argued that nursing is a science, an emerging science, an applied science, an art, or a combination of both art and science. The debate continues but claims that nursing is (or can be) a science are in the majority. It is also a debate which is best understood in the context of several interrelated issues: (1) nursing is an occupation which is professionalising an extension of traditional female roles in which caring is central but poorly valued; (2) science has a dominant and valued place in our society, and nurses have attempted to improve their status by scientising their knowledge base; (3) nurses have acknowledged that their work has been undervalued and relatively invisible; and (4) nurses have had a long fight for better education and knowledge.

Nursing's quest for scientific status has been a difficult one, not only because most nurses are women and they have been poorly educated, but also because nursing is an area of women's work, it is poorly valued, and nursing education has been poorly funded, and because there is a limit to the extent to which nursing practice can fit with dominant views of science. That has not stopped nurses (and others who study nurses and nursing), however, from attempting to articlate nursing reality using ill-fitting models (if only to get research funding), or from taking on methodologies which other disciplines are rejecting as inadequate. Such a process illustrates the extent to which scientific constructions of knowledge have dominated disciplines which are concerned with non-reductive and non-positivist lines of enquiry. Within these constraints, however, nurses have managed to conduct a vast array of studies which have immediate and direct relevance to the care of patients and clients. Such work, however, leaves outside the research process, issues of central relevance to nursing reality – questions such as what it **feels** like to be ill or in pain, or how interpersonal and professional ambience make people feel better or worse and get better more or less quickly. While many nursing issues lend themselves to quantification, measurement and positivist enquiry, such approaches do not encapsulate the whole story, or what one might regard as the things which really matter to the people in question.

Silva and Rothbart (1984:7–8) argue that nursing began to embrace logical empiricism in the 1960s at a time when the limitations of this approach were becoming apparent to philosophers of science. Gortner (1983:4) explains, however, that lack of doctoral programs in nursing meant that nurses acquired their research training in disciplines other than nursing and, as a consequence, they took on the paradigms of those disciplines, applied them to nursing, and conducted controlled experimental work – a process exacerbated by funding agencies which preferred controlled studies. As a result of this and other things, nursing research has been predominantly empiricist, though, the trend is moving more toward phenomenological and existential works, particularly since the 1980s. The strange paradox, however, is that theory development and empirical work have tended to be relatively independent of each other (Silva & Rothbart 1984) – theory development has (in the main) emphasised holism and the research has been predominantly empiricist and positivist.

The relative independence of theory and research is mirrored by a similar mis-match between ideology (philosophy) and methodology (Winstead-Fry 1980, Munhall 1982b, Tinkle & Beaton 1983). While research has been predominantly empiricist, nursing theory has been the product (mostly) of nurses intellectualising, contemplating and philosophising their practice. And although nursing ideology has continued to stress holism and humanistic values, its methodologies have been predominantly objective and reductive. There are two concepts which evolved from attempts to scientise practice, the nursing process and the metaparadigm of nursing, which illustrate the paradoxes.

The nursing process

The nursing process has been espoused as a way, if not **the** way, to scientise nursing (see, for example, Mauksch & David 1972, Humphris 1979, La Monica 1979:xiii, Marriner 1983) by assessing patients' needs using nursing histories (a term adapted from medicine), writing a plan of care (documentation is stressed), implementing that care and then evaluating it. More recently, another step was added – making nursing diagnoses (another term adapted from medicine).

The limitations of the nursing process are now being recognised and criticisms of it are growing. It is seen as denigrating the knowledge which is derived from experience because it excludes ways of knowing that are non-logistic (Henderson 1982), can be used as an instrument of authority (Donnelly 1987), and does not take account of the knowledge of expert practitioners (McHugh 1986:26–27), and there has been persistent resistance among registered nurses to having this concept of practice imposed upon them. They see it as unnecessary paper work, which requires them to write down what is, to them, obvious and self-evident, e.g. the 'need' for a daily wash. The real irony, however, is that although the nursing process is promoted as a tool to enhance holistic and humanistic practice, it is positivist, reductive and mechanistic, to the extent that the patient is, or can be, reduced (at least on paper) to set of problems, needs, or diagnoses. It is an approach to practice which mimics medicine and positivist methodologies, and it is inadequate if we are to accommodate lived body experience (Parker 1988, Gadow 1980, 1982, Benner & Wrubel 1988). Use of the nursing process, which involves taking a nursing history, also poses a danger of subjecting the patient to what could be called a 'nursing gaze' – to adapt a term from Foucault (1976). In the quest to document patients' needs and make nursing diagnoses, there is potential for the patient to be the subject of unnecessary surveillance, about which more will be said in Chapter 2.

The nursing metaparadigm

The metaparadigm of nursing is said to consist of the four concepts of nursing, health, environment, and man (later amended to person). These four concepts are seen as fundamental in organising the concerns of the discipline, and they have been accepted, particularly among American nurses, who are said to be in consensus on the issue (see Fawcett 1984, Flaskerud & Halloran 1980). Nonetheless, there are critics of the notion that nursing has a metaparadigm. Brodie (1984), for example, has suggested that the metaparadigm should be seen more as a stage nursing is going through rather than a definitive statement about the discipline or its future directions.

As a worst case scenario, the metaparadigm has the potential to restrict nursing theory development, and Brodie (1984) has urged caution about the possibilities of foreclosing on interesting and creative concepts, especially those derived from research. However, although support for the metaparadigm is said to be drawn from the research literature, at least in part, that research literature is itself a problem because it has been predominantly empiricist.

There is an added complication that, even though the metaparadigm is so broad it can potentially accommodate anything, it does not reflect research questions which can be posed outside mainstream positivist science. The metaparadigm, however, has already become an important organising framework. Several textbooks have used it to structure material (see, for example, Fitzpatrick & Whall 1983), and it has become the international cataloguing system for doctoral theses, where, incidentally, it has given rise to some strange indexing.

The metaparadigm can also be seen as a reflection of nursing's attempts to be seen as a discipline with a developed knowledge base and concepts unique to itself. The metaparadigm, however, is apparently inclusive at the same time as it excludes some things. Where, for instance, could it accommodate the body, and how would it be used to categorise this study?

Most of the empirical literature which concerns the body focuses on what Goddard (1953, cited by Melia 1979) called 'technical nursing' and it is a rapidly expanding literature. This material deals with technological aspects of care which stem from the application of new equipment, new procedures in medicine and better understanding of physiology and biochemistry. It is neither material which concerns 'dirt' nor material which reflects existential aspects of embodiment, and about which nurses are concerned in their daily practice. If the metaparadigm is a reflection of what is reserached, there is an inherent problem generated by the social and institutional infrastructures which influence why some things are researched and others remain silent. The metaparadigm may only tell us what is being researched and not what the central concerns of nursing are in practice. It does not, for example, explicitly acknowledge the body either in its object sense or in relation to embodied existence.

THE BODY AND BODY CARE IN NURSING TEXTS

What literature there is on 'basic nursing' (physical body care) is almost exclusively recipe-type procedural material which emphasises how to do certain tasks and it contains information derived from tradition and experience, not research. Such material forms a substantial part of any text on nursing care, and it is from those texts that one can deduce something of the manner in which the body and body care, have been conceptualised and taught in formal nursing education[1].

Textbooks for nurses can generally be divided into three groups. The first group includes those which are essentially manuals which outline how to perform various nursing procedures, including the necessary related equipment and any particular precautions or associated dangers. The second group includes books written by medical practitioners specifically for nurses, and these consist of condensed and abbreviated medical knowledge – what medical practitioners think nurses need to know, at least from their viewpoint. The third and most recent category of texts are those written by nurses which are comprehensive in their approach, integrating theoretical and empirical material with instructions on nursing procedures. There are also some 'mixed' texts and those which deal with specific topics which do not fit neatly into any of these major categories, though, because they are not centrally concerned with body care, they will not be discussed here.

Each category of texts has a particular style of conceptualising the body, but it is the first and third groups that I want to examine here. Those written by medical practitioners (the second category of texts) take a characteristic medical approach to the body in emphasising disease manifestations and medical treatment. Except for illustrating the medical approach to the body (which has already been discussed), they usually do not provide instructional material about body management in nursing practice, in contrast to those written by nurses.

The first group of texts must be examined in its historical context, because this was the original written material for nurse education and elements of the approach they promoted continue in current texts and educational practices (see Lawler 1984). In addition, many of the interviewees in this study would have used such texts as prescribed reading as students, and their professional competence (when they were students) would have been assessed against the standards set down in the texts of the day.

Texts on nursing procedures

The material in these books consists of directions on how to perform the vast array of nursing procedures and therapeutics – washing people, applying splints and bandages, dressings, administering enemas and the like. Such books were invariably written by nurses, but they generally included input from medical practitioners. The subject matter they contain overwhelmingly concerns the body and how to deal with those things which nurses need to do for dependent patients. There is usually also a moderate amount of material dealing with relationships among colleagues, including the medical practitioner, and inevitably material on how the nurse should conduct herself [sic] professionally both giving patient care and in her private life. Additionally, there is usually instruction on what could be called domestic matters, for example, keeping the ward environment clean and tidy, and in some cases, recipes for preparing special food for the sick – 'invalid cookery'.

A typical example of this type of text is Burbidge's (1935)

Lectures for Nurses. It includes notes on procedural things as well as material on anatomy and physiology, common cures of the day, and ethics, and she implied that the nurse has some sort of special responsibility to avoid suspicion about her 'character'. While reference to 'character' may have been a result of the poor reputation of nurses in the previous century (see Abel-Smith 1977), which still lingers, there is the suggestion that nursing work has features which must be delicately managed. She advises the reader to 'cultivate a good professional manner, [to be] efficient, but not officious. Be dignified, unflurried, cheerful and unfailingly courteous' (Burbidge 1935:11–12). In addition the nurse is urged to consider that 'the peculiarly intimate character of a nurse's contact with her [sic] patients demands a well balanced personality . . .' (1935:12).

Texts like those of Burbidge's seldom mention anything, except for references to a 'professional manner', which one could identify as social methods to help in the management of other people's bodies. The language and style were invariably detached, clinical, procedural and objective, the emphasis being starkly on the object body, and the body as object. There is little, if any, discussion of what one could call the experiential aspects of doing nursing procedures or being the recipient of them. These texts, however, reflect the linguistic style of other texts (see, for example, *Mrs Beeton's Book of Household Management*, first published in 1859) about matters relating to traditional women's work, including nursing, which evolved as an extension of domestic service.

However, the paradoxical approach to the importance of body care, which seems to pervade nursing, is obvious in the early texts, and so too is the recognition that the body is part of lived experience. There is constant reference in Burbidge's (1935) book to the need to ensure that the patient is not unduly exposed, and for the procedure to be done conscientiously. This material is, however, introduced early in the book, and typically it is material taught early in students' training, where it is established as 'introductory' concepts and skills, but with the added notion that such things are fundamental. The language is heavily imbued with what the nurse 'must' and 'should' do, but what reference there is to social management is characterised by coyness. While these features reflect the strictness which typified nursing education, as well as general social attitudes, they nevertheless indicate a certain taken-for-granted approach to the body and what nurses must do to it in nursing care.

The Burbidge text provides a description of how the nurse should do an 'Admission Sponge'. This is a useful example because, as the later Chapters will show, sponging is the centrepiece of body care. The language which Burbidge used is particularly frank, but is also typically procedural, objective, if not objectifying and clinical.

Method – Remove the top bedclothes, leaving the patient covered with the old blanket. Remove the clothes, folding them neatly and placing them on a chair at the side of the bed, ready to deal with them as soon as the sponge is finished.

Do not unduly expose the patient while sponging. Watch carefully for any abnormality, bruising, burns, redness, rash, discharges, et cetera, and report the matter to sister.

Wash and dry face and ears first, then each hand and arm, paying particular attention to each axilla (armpit). Using second face washer, sponge chest. When dealing with stout women, be particularly watchful for any sore areas under the breasts. Then wash abdomen. Be sure the umbilicus (navel) is quite clean.

Change water. Sponge each leg. Wash and dry well between the toes. Cut the toe nails. Gently turn, wash back and buttocks. Put on one-half of the bedgown, roll the under blanket towards the centre of the bed. Turn patient on to the other side of the bed, remove under blanket, and finish putting on the bedgown. Wash in the region of the groin. This is to be done under cover of a towel, so that the patient need not be embarrassed. Discriminate between prudery and refinement. Remember that as the nurse you are responsible for the scrupulous cleanliness of the patient.

Replace upper bedclothes over the patient, removing the second old blanket. Pleats are made in the sheet and blankets at the foot of the bed, and the quilt (without pleats) is replaced. Manicure finger nails. Place towel over pillow, comb and fine comb hair (tact is very necessary in regard to this), report condition of the hair in the Head Book.

See that the patient is warm and comfortable. Clear everything away from the bedside, seeing that the locker is within reach, and the chair is in line with the top of the bed. Move screen last of all (Burbidge 1935:22–23).

The linguistic style of this account does not differ essentially from the directions that would be provided in a recipe for making a cake. It is directive and objectifying, and it is reductive. Body care is a set procedure, and the patient – the object of this procedure – is fundamentally a body, albeit one with the potential for feelings. From a world view located in the 1990s the approach suggested by Burbidge seems particularly detached and objectifying. It is likely, however, that such a manner was necessary as a means of dealing with the taboos associated with the body in an era when fewer areas of the body were exposed and nakedness was rare. Being able to focus on the procedure is one way that the nurse could overcome a highly invasive act, and some of those I spoke with in this study admit to managing some socially awkward procedures in this way.

In later decades of this century, however, we have become accustomed to such things as nude bathing, and exposure of the body is an everyday occurrence on film and television. It is another matter entirely, though, to be involved with nakedness of other people in the kind of situations nurses must manage as novices.

A more recent text than Burbidge's, and one which enjoyed such wide and popular use that it is a classic in Australian nursing education, is Doherty, Sirl and Ring's *Modern Practical Nursing Procedures* (1965). Originally published in 1944, and 'recommended by the N.S.W. Nurses' Registration Board for adoption by training schools preparing student nurses . . .' (1965:ix), this text was reprinted on many occasions and was still in wide use until the 1970s. This text shows signs of attempting to locate the procedures nurses perform in a more person-oriented context. The 1965 edition, for example, starts with a chapter on communication and encourages the nurse to 'develop skill of communication by learning to talk **with** the patient, not to or at him [sic]' (1965:1) and it emphasises the various ways in which messages can be communicated to patients. The second chapter, however, concerns 'Ethics and Hospital Etiquette', and there is the typical inclusion of material on domestic matters. There is also an increasing emphasis on what Goddard (1953, cited in Melia 1979) called 'technical nursing', which reflected developments in science, technology, and medicine.

The body care material in the Doherty et al text shows no real differences from those in the Burbidge text described above, except that the language is less recipe-like, and there is more specific language than that which Burbidge used with respect to parts of the body. For example, where Burbidge (1935:23) had directed the nurse to 'wash in the region of the groin' Doherty et al (1965:55) are more explicit and state that 'the external genital area is carefully washed and dried. The patient usually prefers to wash this area himself [sic] but must be assisted by the nurse if necessary'.

Another standard and classic text in Australian nursing was Smith and Lew's *Nursing Care of the Patient* (1975). It was first published in 1968 and was widely used well into the early 1980s. It is similar in many ways to the Doherty et al text, except that Smith and Lew show the influence of a needs-based approach to care – a trend which was eventually embodied in 'the nursing process', in which assessment of the patient's needs is integral.

While the linguistic style of Smith and Lew (1975, see especially Ch. 13) is not as directive and objectifying, there is a similar set of step-wise instructions about how one conducts body care for others.

In the chapter entitled 'Making the Patient Comfortable', the nurse is urged by the authors to consider the psychological aspects of patient care and comfort, but it is essentially advice on ways the nurse can be kind to patients. There is no recognisable material on the social management of nursing care, rather, only the procedural material. Embedded in the style of the text, however, is an implied assumption that if the nurse takes notice of the advice, 'her' [sic] job will be done better, and patients will be co-operative or compliant. There is no suggestion that the patient may object to any of the procedures which are described. It is taken for granted that patients are compliant – a theme which is discussed in a later chapter of this book.

Comprehensive and empirically based texts

More recently, texts such as those described above have been supplanted by those which I categorise as comprehensive and empirically based. A well established text of this kind is Henderson and Nite's *Principles and Practice of Nursing* (1978), a book which is stylistically typical of those in common usage in academic nursing and health occupations today. Although editions of this book have been published since the 1950s, their scope, style and content would not have suited the hospital-based programs that existed for the training of nurses in this country. Therefore, there is a limit to the influence such work would have had in the Australian context until the 1980s, and most nurses in this study were educated prior to that time. These books are useful, though, to analyse because of what they illustrate. The Henderson and Nite text, like most of the comprehensive type, emanates from North America, while the three books discussed earlier were all published in Australia by authors whose professional traditions (and therefore cultural traditions) would have a substantial British influence. Such differences are important in dealing with the body because of the cultural variations in taboos about, and ways of dealing with, the body.

The Henderson and Nite (1978) text takes an explicit and direct approach to the business of basic body care. In contrast to the texts which are almost exclusively procedure manuals, Henderson and Nite acknowledge the social difficulties of dealing with other people's bodies. For example, they say that washing a patient in bed may

involve an exposure of the body to which many persons are unaccustomed. Exposure of the genitalia is probably the chief cause of discomfort. When patients' conditions permit, they bathe the genital-anal region themselves, but nurses must be prepared and willing to give this service. Because in almost all cultures the genitalia are covered, exposure of the pudenda is embarrassing to most persons. The extent to which so-called modesty is innate or acquired is the subject of endless discussion. Health practices should be based on the assumption that, whether innate or acquired, the exposure of the genitalia is distasteful to many if not most persons. Having the genitalia touched is an even greater infringement of privacy and it may elicit an erotic response. In the boy or man there may be an erection of the penis. But in spite of these consequences it is obvious that help must be given some persons in keeping the genitalia clean . . . (Henderson & Nite 1978:787).

The section on physical care goes on to describe why it is important to ensure good body hygiene and draws extensively on the research literature for rationales in support of various practices. It is in stark contrast to the recipe book approach of other texts, although the same emphasis is placed on the need to be kind, and to follow a procedure whereby one starts to wash from the head and works down toward the more 'dirty' parts of the body. There are also explicit directions on how to wash the genitalia (1978:792), rather than simply stating, as Burbidge (1935:23) did, to 'wash in the region of the groin'. One interesting aspect of the procedures outlined by Henderson and Nite (1978:792) is the suggestion that the nurse might wear disposable gloves for washing the genitalia. It is not made explicit, however, if this is for aesthetic or hygiene related reasons, or some other reason(s).

So, while some information about the ways nurses have conceptualised the body care which is integral to their job, can be gleaned from an analysis of some typical textbooks,[2] we have only a limited picture of how nurses' work with the body fits into a social framework. There is some literature in this field, and in the main, the principal points of reference are the notions that nursing is dirty work, and that it is women's work.

DIRTY WORK AND NURSING

Dirty work is not a well studied subject, but one of the earliest and most important writers on the topic was Everett Hughes. He was also one of the earliest to write about the sociology of nursing in his essay, 'Studying the Nurse's Work', which he first published in 1951 (1971). He did not, however, define what he meant by the term 'dirty work', rather he used it as a taken-for-granted notion about a moral division of labour.

Constructs of dirty work

In his paper on the persecution of Jews and others in Nazi Germany during the Hitler regime, Hughes (1971) suggests that those who do dirty work are acting as agents for the rest of society by doing dirty work that others will not do, but which they require or desire to be done for them. Dirty workers, he argues, are integral to any society. He also suggests it is possible that dirty workers are in some way psychologically warped and that, for those people, there is some attraction in dirty work. He was, however, influenced by the extent to which 'normal' Germans went on with life, tacitly condoning the murder of Jews. His explanations, which focus on the psychology of the individual as well as their agency role in social life, were criticised by Davis (1984), who suggests that Hughes' position can serve as a distancing mechanism for the 'good' people, who have others do their dirty work for them. He further argues that we 'should consider the possibility that many dirty workers are really no different from the good people; that they are good people *doing* dirty work' (Davis 1984:234)

As social scientists have tried to capture the social functions of dirty work and the effects of such work on those who do it, the picture has not become much clearer. Hughes, for example, was working in the immediate post-war period, when gross social upheaval was beyond the experience of many of those who studied it, and in Hughes' work on Nazi Germany we can identify an attempt to conceptualise dirty work on the scale of grand theory, integrating both social structural and functional (though not functionalist) elements with the psychological. Most of the literature on dirty work seems to be of this ilk, where the researchers have attempted to illustrate the effects on those who do work designated as dirty, and they have explored the social meaning of the work itself. The data reported from my study are similar because it is not sufficient only to plot the mechanisms which 'dirty workers' use to manage their work, but one must also explore what it is in society that gives rise to a need for dirty work to be managed at all.

In his essay on 'Work and Self' Hughes (1971:343–344) argues that all occupations have some level of dirty work, and that the dirty work must be dealt with in some way, either by concealment, delegation to someone of lower status, or, when the potential for delegation is limited, by being integrated into the total context of an occupation. Each of these mechanisms operates to some extent in nursing. In the more traditional system of assigning tasks rather than patients, nurses assign dirty work associated with the body to low status staff. They also use concealment by doing much of their dirty jobs behind closed doors or behind screens (which they see as maintaining the patient's privacy). And they integrate body care into the job, especially in the more recent forms of division of labour where one nurse has responsibility for the entire nursing care of a particular patient or group of patients (so-called 'total patient care'). The mechanism of concealment is, however, the most difficult to study, because by its very nature it tends to make the work invisible or inaccessible to the researcher.

Bailbondsmen are socially isolated because of their work and they contribute to that isolation themselves (Davis 1984). Many of them are aware that they are engaged in a low status occupation, which is also stigmatised, and that the social isolation they face is partly a result of the nature of their work. Concealment of dirty work, as Hughes described it, also operates to remove from the public arena that which is designated as dirty (see also Davis 1984). What is designated dirty is also invisible and taboo. So there is a strong link between dirty work and taboo subjects, and much of the work that nurses do is both dirty and taboo, and it is largely invisible.

Emerson and Pollner (1976), however, have argued that dirty work is a function of perspective. They claim that it is not sufficient to talk only in terms of 'dirty work', but also in terms of 'dirty work designations' (1976:243–244). This is because dirtiness does not inhere in the task but that 'something of the judger is involved in the judgement, as dirty work designations are not merely the verbal mirrors of a task's inherent qualities' (Emerson & Pollner 1976:244). They further claim that such designations, while being the product of a particular perspective . . . are also the means through which the perspective is enacted and perpetuated' (1976:244). They are, therefore, arguing for an interpretive and interactive viewpoint for examining dirty work.

Emerson and Pollner (1976) also argue that, at least in so far as community mental health care is concerned, practitioners are more likely to regard as dirty those jobs where they can achieve little. This also holds for general medical practitioners who have to treat alcoholics (Strong 1980), and for certain categories of casualty patients (Jeffrey 1979). Dirty work in general nursing, although sharing many of the features of other kinds of dirty work, is different to the extent that the body care nurses do, not only constitutes a moral division of labour, in Hughes' (1971) terms, but in a very real sense it is also potentially inherently dirty. Nurses in the study reported here, however, did not link their dirty work to potential for achievement, as was the case in the studies of Strong (1980), Emerson and Pollner (1976), or Jeffrey (1979). For example, although the dying patient requires increasingly more time for body care, and health care is predominantly cure-oriented, nurses see what they do as more important as the dying patient moves progressively closer to death. In a curative sense they achieve nothing, but such a perspective of achieving nothing is meaningful only in the context of a social environment where death is a failure to cure. To nurses, care of the dying is seen within an entirely different perspective.

Nursing as dirty work

What studies there have been done on nurses' work reveal a highly consistent viewpoint that, in part, it is designated dirty work, especially that which involves direct contact with the body or body products. Stannard (1973) studied patient care and abuse in a nursing home and found that body care, and care for the elderly generally, were regarded as low status work, done by people of low social status, or those with 'spoiled identities' (after Goffman 1981). Their work was also concealed from public view.

In a more recent study, Wolf (1986a, 1986b) argues that nurses' dirty work is a case of the sacred and profane. Nurses work brings them into 'direct contact with bodily products, including secretions and excretions, and with the products of infection' (1986a:29), and it has been made socially manageable historically through an association with religion and ritual. She further argues that there has been an historical link between dirty work and the belief that, because women were considered unclean, particularly during menstruation, they were ideal for such work (1986a). While women were supposedly suited to this work, and while the work itself was recognised as dirty, there was a concomitant emphasis on the need not only for personal cleanliness on the part of the nurse, but also for her to remain morally pure. This would seem to suggest a fear about the nature of the work that nurses do, and ample evidence can also be found to show that nursing has incorporated professional traditions drawn from religion and from religious orders (Wolf 1986a), which also have associations with the control of taboos and culturally defined fears (Colliere 1986).

Nurses have been aware, too, that what they do as work, especially body care, is sometimes repugnant to others. Fagin and Diers (1984:16) describe some typical examples:

For some time now we have been curious about the reactions of people we meet socially to being told. 'I am a nurse'. First reactions to this statement include the comment, 'I never met a nurse socially before'; stories about a person's latest hospitalization, surgery, or childbearing experiences; the question 'How can you bear handling bedpans (vomit, blood)?' or the remark, 'I think I need another drink'. We believe the statements reflect the fact that nursing evokes disturbing and discomforting images that many educated, middle-class, upwardly mobile Americans find difficult to handle in a social situation.

They suggest that the work and roles of nurses can be seen as a metaphor for many things including the following: motherhood, because the nurse does for the patient similar things that a mother (parent) does for a child; equality, because in the nurse-patient relationship the class of the patient is largely irrelevant; and intimacy, because 'nurses do for others publicly what healthy persons do for themselves behind closed doors' (Fagin & Diers 1984:16). Nursing is a metaphor for sex because

having seen and touched the bodies of strangers, nurses are perceived as willing and able sexual partners. Knowing and experienced, they, unlike prostitutes, are thought to be safe – a quality suggested by the cleanliness of their white uniforms and their professional aplomb (Fagin & Diers 1984:17).

Other works on the nature, content, and context of nurses' work illustrate the difficulty of developing an accurate picture of what nurses do, and this is especially true of body care. Webster's (1985) study of medical students' views on the role of nurses shows that what nurses do is not readily available to the public gaze, not even to medical students who share the same clinical environment. In Webster's (1985:315) study, first and second year male students were more likely than either female students or students in more advanced years to see nurses as 'scut workers', i.e. those who do the cleaning up and cleaning of patients, as well as other tasks which the medical student believed to be of low status. Female students were more accurately informed, it seemed, because many of them had shared accommodation with nursing students. Although the people in Webster's sample believed they had a good grasp of what nurses did, they became increasingly vague about the specifics as they progressed through their course, especially with respect to the interface between medicine and nursing.

Two Australian studies are worth particular mention. The first of these, by Wilson and Najman (1982), neither of whom is a nurse, was conducted in Queensland using a sample of 548 open-ended questionnaires from anonymous participants. They detail a large number of nursing activities, leading the researchers to comment that 'the range of knowledge which a nurse is apparently expected to provide is astonishing' (Wilson & Najman 1982:32). However, in this 'astonishing' list, there is no mention of body care.

The second study, by Bonawit and Whittaker (1983), both of whom are nurses, was conducted in Victoria. They wanted to document the knowledge, attitudes, and beliefs about nursing behaviours among a sample of 250 nurses and 250 non-nurses. They plotted levels of congruence in beliefs between the nurses and non-nurses for various nursing functions, which the researchers listed. They concluded that there was 'no significant difference in knowledge of what nurses do between the two groups of respondents in areas related to generally well defined nursing functions, for example, washing patients, giving medications, dressing wounds, taking vital signs and giving first aid' (Bonawit & Whittaker 1983:52), that is, doing what Goddard (1953, cited by Melia 1979) called 'basic nursing'. The authors also conclude that there was a lack of knowledge among the non-nurses about the extent to which nursing was an occupation with autonomous functions independent of, or commonly ascribed to, medical practitioners. Historically, however, nursing has been regarded as an occupation subservient to, and dependent on, medicine – a relationship with men's work which defines nursing as women's work in a gendered division of labour.

WOMEN'S WORK AND NURSING

Power (1975:226) has summarised women's work as that which replicates 'women's household functions and/or household sex relationships', where the majority of workers are women, where men are in authority over the work that women do, especially 'work associated with food, clothing and cleaning and work which involves caring for the young and the sick' (1975:227–228), and where there is the associated belief that this is all 'natural'. In such a framework as Power's, nursing is prototypically women's work.

Nursing is a highly sex-typed female occupation with a history of having been dominated and controlled by a male medical profession (Willis 1979, 1983). In its modern (post-Nightingale) form it grew out of a background association with domestic service (see Abel-Smith 1977), and there has been the strongly held belief that nursing skills were a refinement of the 'natural' (biologically determined) talents of women (Gamarnikow 1978:98–99). Additionally, nursing has all four of the characteristic features of the role of housewife which Oakley (1982:1) identified – '*exclusive allocation to women*, rather than to adults of both sexes; . . . association with *economic dependence*, . . . *status as non-work* – or its opposition to 'real' work, i.e. economically productive work, and . . . *primacy* to women, that is, . . . priority over other roles'.

In social and economic terms nursing falls between the public and the private. Nurses operate in the public arena in doing paid labour, yet their work is heavily dictated by what would normally be the private, and therefore, unpaid, domain for healthy people. Nursing work represents a transformation of the (normally) private to the public, but traditionally payment for such work been has been low, and the occupation has not enjoyed high status. The usual explanation is that nursing is essentially a form of women's work and, therefore, it simply reflects women's work in general.[3]

The central assumption which cements together ideas and stereotypes about women's work, and nursing in particular, is the belief in a biological suitability of women to some work. This is clearly demonstrated, for example, in Bennett's (1984) study of decisions of the Australian Conciliation and Arbitration Court 1907–1921, when crucial principles were established about men's work and women's work. She argues that while we may emphasise the political, social, and economic processes which sustain a sexual division of labour, the idea that women and men are biologically different, and therefore suited to different work, has not been strongly challenged.

Biological determinism has been a mainstay in the construction of nursing as women's work (Gamarnikow 1978). The central idea is that one firstly has to be a 'good woman' in order to be a 'good' nurse. Gamarnikow cites extensively from original Nightingale writings to summarise the ideological background in which the occupation of nursing took on its modern form.

Nightingale insisted on the existence of a close link between nursing and femininity, the latter being defined by a specific combination of moral qualities which differentiated men from women. The success of nursing reforms depended primarily, according to Nightingale, on cultivating the 'feminine' character, rather than on training and education (Gamarnikow 1978:116).

As well as the beliefs about the innate abilities of women which suited them to the role of nurse, Gamarnikow (1978) details the close historical connections between the organisation of nursing and division of labour within it. The organisation of nursing work was an extension and a mirror of major households, complete with a strict hierarchy of people and the tasks they performed. What transformed nursing, however, into something different from just another variation of the Victorian household, was an adherence to the idea that nursing was the science of hygiene. However, Gamarnikow (1978:118) argues that one consequence of this was that most of the domestic work in hospitals was allocated to nurses – a situation which was subsequently changed, but only recently.

While nurses may have relinquished their responsibility for such domestic affairs as cleaning rooms and the patients' physical surroundings, they have retained those parts of domesticity that have to do with the sanitary aspects of patient care. Herein lies one of the essential difficulties for examining nursing from the viewpoint only of women's work. It is not sufficient to see nursing only in terms of its links to traditional domestic and household roles associated with women because consideration must be given to the body in nurses' work. Caring for the bodies of others must take account of two elements – caring, which is strongly associated with women, and the body. The body has an association with women to the extent that much of their work indirectly concerns the body, for example, washing clothes, cooking and cleaning; and in mothering there is a need to care for the bodies of children. In nursing, however, the body is an explicit and direct focus of attention, and it is work conducted outside the context of family life.[4]

Lewin (1977:79) observed that 'nursing work hovers perilously close to the traditional nurturance and submission which feminists have shown to be related to the oppression of women' because the very nature of nursing centres on doing for others in the same way that a mother (and more recently perhaps also a father) would do for a child.

The identification of nursing with femaleness derives not only from its 'unselfish service' component, but from the importance of physical nurturance, and a sort of material intimacy, which also enter into the image of nursing work. The close acquaintance of the nurse with the messy private details of illness is not unlike the mother's necessary involvement with infantile body functions (Lewin 1977:91).

Lewin has summarised the position of nursing well in highlighting a relationship between women's work, the body, and dirty work. These three characteristics, individually and collectively, come together in the context of the occupation of nursing. The chapters which follow attempt to construct an understanding of how the body is dealt with in the social sciences and society and how nurses socially manage their work and integrate it into everyday life.

NOTES

1. It is important to make a distinction between 'formal' (classroom) education and 'informal' education (that which is learned on the job) in nursing. While nurses are instructed in those matters which are contained in textbooks, there is sometimes considerable dislocation between that knowledge and what is learned in clinical practice (see Lawler 1984).

2. Some other examples of comprehensive texts can be found in other texts. For example:

   Beverly Du Gas' *Introduction to Patient Care* (published in 1983 by Saunders, Philadelphia) has a less didactic style when body care is described and she emphasises the opportunities body care procedures provide for the nurse to get to know the patient better. However, although the rationale for body care is explained in detail, there is the usual list of recipe-like steps the nurse could use in carrying out the procedure.

   Malinda Murray's *Fundamentals of Nursing* (published in 1980 by Prentice-Hall, Englewood Cliffs) uses an approach similar to that used by Du Gas, but in addition she makes special mention of the embarrassment that washing the genital area may induce for the patient. No information is given, however, in how this might be managed other than to avoid unnecessary exposure of, for example, the breasts of women.

   M.D. Emerton's *Principles and Practice of Nursing* (published in 1980 by University of Queensland Press, St. Lucia) (see in particular, pp.71–75) is another example of the typical recipe book approach to body care.

   Bernadette Ibell's *Integrated Basic Theory and Practice of Nursing* (published in 1979 by Pitman Medical Australia, Carlton) describes body care procedures in a style which incorporates much advice and what could be called 'tricks of the trade' about how to manage the technical aspects of the procedure. For example, (on page 389) she advises the nurse not to 'screw the washer up into a tiny ball, but . . . [that it should be] held firmly in . . . [the nurse's] hand'. There is not mention of managing the social aspects of this procedure except for the usual reference to privacy.

   B. Kozier and G. Erb's *Fundamentals of Nursing: Concepts and Products* (published in 1983 by Addison-Wesly, Menlo Park) uses the familiar procedural approach to body care, but they have added detailed rationales for aspects of body care in an apparent attempt to scientise them.

3. One cannot discount, however, works such as those of Ehrenreich and English (1976) and Shorter (1984) which show how our cultural heritage is typified by mystifing and fearing the power of women's bodies and women's perceived privileged knowledge of bodies. Women's knowledge of bodies was also a source of power which men, in particular, sought to control. One consequence of this process of control was a division of labour over the body between medicine (men) and nursing (women) which resulted in the low status work on the body being assigned to nurses and the high status aspects becoming the province of medical practitioners. While it is possible to trace these historical links, this whole debate is often complicated by what could be regarded as irrational fears of women and unfounded notions about women which emanate from the power of women's bodies (see Chesler 1978) and the knowledge which women have of bodily things.

4. Within the family setting, however, women's traditional roles include

responsibility for the care and comfort of sick family members and nursing's historical links to the home work of women in this respect is well established. What is not well established as a primary focus of discussion is women's role, directly and indirectly, in the care and maintenance of the bodies of others, though the considerable literature on women's unpaid domestic labour has inferred this to be the case. Domestic labour has subsumed work related to the body, but the body itself, as a central point of discussion has been present by implication in such things as cleaning, washing and the doing of housework.

2. Conceptualising the body

This chapter will start to trace the literature from which an understanding of the body in social life can be constructed. This is done, firstly, by examining how the body has been conceptualised in philosophy, and how the body has changed in social history and in relation to society and the state, and secondly, by discussing the place of the body in sociology and social theory.

PHILOSOPHISING THE BODY

Descartes was one of the earliest philosophers to write about 'the problem of the (human) body' and he is often, although wrongly, attributed with having originated the conceptual split between mind and body. He recognised the metaphysical difficulty in both having and being a body, of being both the substance of, and existent in, the same entity. It was a difficulty he did not resolve, rather, centuries later we hear of so-called 'Cartesian dualism' – the view that mind and body are separate. However, Descartes (1986:159) had acknowledged, in his Sixth Meditation, that mind and body were interdependent, observing that

> nature ... teaches me by ... feelings of pain, hunger, thirst, etc. that I am not only lodged in my body like a pilot in his ship, but, besides, that I am joined to it very closely and indeed so compounded and intermingled with my body, that I form, as it were, a single whole with it.

What Descartes was acknowledging here was not some objective and measurable reality of the body, but a body which was understood through his own experience and practical knowledge. It is not the sort of knowledge typical of disciplines which study the body *or* the mind because they overlook practical knowledge and experience in favour of knowledge which is less holistic, more positivist and which lends itself to scientising, reduction and objectification. What

Descartes described is more typical of disciplines which rely on the experience of being human, such as drama, music, and nursing and which cannot be explored (easily or comfortably) within a dominant logico-positivist construction of knowledge. We have, however, a configuration of knowledges built around dualisms, of which the Cartesian variety (so-called) is one.

Historically, disciplines have not dealt with the problem of the mind **and** the body, as Descartes had done, but with the mind **or** the body. Philosophy has usually been concerned with the former (Harre 1986, Rothfield 1986) and social scientists have also largely ignored the latter (Turner 1984, Rothfield 1986, Caddick 1986). Those who have dealt with non-body topics have largely ignored emotions except in their negative sense (Hochschild 1975), although Kemper (1978) attempted a sociology of emotions which addressed physiological processes. Recently, however, the body has become increasingly popular as an area of study in social science (see, for example, Scott 1981, Scarry 1985, O'Neill 1986, Kroker & Kroker 1988a, Shalom 1989), and it is becoming especially important for feminism (see, in particular, Kristeva 1982, Rothfield 1986, Caddick 1986, Suleiman 1986, Australian Feminist Studies (5) 1987, Gatens 1988, Irigaray 1987, Ussher 1989, Martin 1987, Jaggar & Bordo 1989).

The body and personhood

Our understanding of the body is firmly interwoven with the nature of personhood[1] and with the meaning of being human, and our notion of human existence requires a bodily form that is recognisable as human. We are human to the extent that we have a physical appearance like that of other humans. To be a human person is also to have a living body (Long 1970:123–125).

Cross-culturally, however, constructions of personhood differ significantly (de Craemer 1983). In the American context, which shares a considerable commonality with other English speaking western countries, personhood is highly individualistic and it is expressed in terms of individual rights (including the right to self-determination), autonomy and privacy (de Craemer 1983:20). According to de Craemer (1983:20), personhood is 'both implicitly and explicitly ... a social and interactive conception of ... human[s]'. He further explains that

The American view of the human person is pervaded by logical-rational dichotomies. This view sharply opposes body and mind, thought and feeling, the conscious and the unconscious, self and other, reality and nonreality (imagining, dreaming, and hearing voices, for example, are not 'real') . . . [and] . . . although it places a high positive value on a universalistic definition of the worth, dignity, and equality of every individual person, it tends to be culturally particularistic, and inadvertently ethnocentric (de Craemer 1983:21).

Neklin (1983) and Fox and Willis (1983) outline how, in practical terms, personhood is a difficult notion to translate into action, especially when it concerns the margins of life – the beginning and the end of life. Questions about when a fetus is sustainable as a separate entity, and how (in this technological era) death is to be defined, hinge on the interface between biology and ethical considerations. The notion of personhood is, therefore, to be considered in a bio-social context because one cannot have personhood without embodiment, and vice versa, if we take social interaction to be a criterion for personhood.

Harre (1986:190) argues that a (human) body is not just another 'thing' because, unlike other things, the person experiences metaphysical ownership of a body in the sense that 'my body' is not 'your body'. And while one 'owns' a body, one also exists in it and experiences it simultaneously. For Harre, an adequate construction of the human body requires integration of the object body-as-thing with the lived body-as-experience. This is consistent with what I have called a somological view of the body, however, most philosophers have emphasised the existential aspects of embodiment, particularly since existentialism became popular.

Jean-Paul Sartre is usually attributed with having opened the modern literature on the existential lived body in his book, *Being and Nothingness* (circa 1960)[2]. Although he was predominantly concerned with the existential self, he wrote about the experience of self as it is mediated by interpersonal and intrapersonal aspects of embodiment. To Sartre, the body is both a being-for-itself (a thing) and a being-for-others (an instrument of and for social interaction). The body-for-itself is perceived by its 'owner' (to take Harre's concept of metaphysical ownership) as a personal sense of embodiment (Sartre circa 1960:304). The body-for-others is the means through which interpersonal interaction becomes possible; a body is a socially defined and constructed instrument which provides an objectification of one person for another (Sartre circa 1960:339) and which can only be perceived in context (Sartre,circa 1960:344). To Sartre (circa 1960:344) personhood and embodiment require each other.

We can not perceive the Other's body *as flesh*, as if it were an isolated object having purely external relations with other thises [things]. That is true only of a *corpse*. The Other's body as flesh is immediately given as the center of reference in a situation which is synthetically organized around it, and it is inseparable from this situation. Therefore we should not ask how the Other's body can be first body for me and subsequently enter into a situation. The Other is originally given to me as a *body in situation*.

In similar terms to Sartre, Merleau-Ponty (1962) emphasised the need to locate the body in context, particularly in time and space, and he argues for the centrality of the body in the development of identity and one's sense of interpersonal being. In this conceptualisation of body and self, Sartre and Merleau-Ponty show the influence of Husserl's existential and phenomenological philosophy in their writings, particularly in their emphasis on the interactive and reflexive nature of the human condition. They acknowledge the role of the body in social encounters among people and within the individual. For Merleau-Ponty (1962:82), one's body is integral to human existence.

The body is the vehicle of being in the world, and having a body is, for a living creature, to be involved in a definite environment, to identify oneself with certain projects and to be continually committed to them (Merleau-Ponty 1962:82).

The body is also a private (intrapersonal) notion of who we are and how we interact with each other, spatially and temporally. For humans, therefore, the qualities of having and being a body are both material and non-material, and, while the body expresses our existence, it cannot be reduced to experience (Merleau-Ponty 1962:166). Yet the philosophical literature reflects a dominant interest in mind as opposed to body, and where the body has been discussed at all it is against a background of human experience, almost as if the philosophers did not know what to do with the object body.

More recently Shalom (1989) has attempted to overcome the artificial split between mind and body by arguing that what it means to be human in terms of experience and embodiment is to be understood through the notion of personal identity. He says that 'the body/mind conceptual framework is an insufficient framework for the task of a philosophical understanding of what we call "the person". That is to say, the concepts "body" and "mind" constitute an insufficient, and therefore misleading, framework...' (1989:403). To Shalom (1989:77) 'body and mind are are what we actually experience as ourselves. They are ourselves as the substance of experiencing'.

The body and medical philosophy

Within medical philosophy, where the object body is a central concern, the work of Erwin Straus is beginning to have an impact on concepts of mind and body as they relate to the experience of illness and medical practice (Cohen 1984, Leder 1984, Pelligrino 1984, Young 1984, Hartmann 1984, Bernal 1984, Williams 1984). The Strausian position criticises the separation of mind and body in medical practice which not only disembodies the person, but which also enables illness to be treated mechanically as pathology of the body. Straus, who is heavily influenced by Merleau-Ponty, emphasises the inherent inter-relationships between mind and body, particularly in matters of illness and in medical encounters. It is in medical encounters or the experience of illness that one is often brought face-to-face with corporeality as part of the human condition. Leder (1984:35) draws on Heidegger's notion of the 'ready-at-hand' to suggest that, in a culture pre-occupied with end use, we only focus on the body when it is not working properly, and that during illness we hand the body over to others for repair and care. 'The problem of the body' is not, therefore, simply abstract and philosophical, it also has personal (interpersonal and intrapersonal), social, sexual, biological, historical and existential dimensions among others, and it requires management to the extent that the body and society are related to each other in a dialectic configuration. This dialectic is poignantly displayed when normal daily life is suspended or interrupted, as it is during illness and hospitalisation, and the body is such a problem that it dominates experience in being a source of discomfort, pain, embarrassment, and vulnerability – all of which require particular management on the part of the patient. In a professional nursing context the dialectic configuration of the body/patient/nurse are central to establishing and maintaining a social order in which care of the most intimate nature is given and received.

THE BODY IN HISTORY

Although it is a physical and organic entity, the human body changes with history. Bodies change over time in relation to social influences on clothing and fashion (Roberts 1977, Colmer 1979, Mullins 1985), culture (see Polhemus 1978, especially Part II A), lifestyle and nutrition (Shorter 1984:Ch. 2). The body is not ahistorical; changes in body shape and size in history illustrate the interface between nature and culture, and between what is represented physically and what that representation symbolises socially. Despite nature, there is a plastic quality to the body, in the sense that it can be moulded to suit different fashions and forms, and one can trace historical trends in the social meanings attached to the body and some of its particular characteristics. The effect of the corset is a prime example, where women's bodies became misshapen to fit a particular kind of ideal body (Colmer 1979, Roberts 1977). What this illustrates is both the historicity of the body, the extent to which individuals' social life and physical form interrelate, and how we have incorporated into our culture the notion that the body is to be controlled and managed. The body in history shows that nature and culture influence each other in these ways.

Some authors (Featherstone 1982, Ableman 1982:25–36, Falk 1985, Lynch 1987) have studied the cultural history in the body, particularly in the ways in which bodies have been moulded to suit culturally determined fashions. Lynch (1987:131) believes that we have come to regard the body as a source of creative expression of the self, a way of expressing individuality and of experiencing personhood, and that 'persons are necessarily corporeal beings' who experience their personhood through their embodiment in an 'historically specific cultural' context. In the Western world of the 1980s and 1990s the culturally specific body form regarded as the ideal type is thin and aerobically fit and it is a body which can be sculpted into a socially defined commodity (Lynch 1987). It would also be reasonable to say that this ideal body is also young and athletic. Such studies as these show how the interface between nature and culture is influenced historically, and they also highlight the need for a theory of the body to accommodate that interface.

THE BODY AND THE STATE

The relationship of the body to the state is probably best understood through the works of Michel Foucault. His analyses illustrate the extent to which the body is an integral part of social life, not only at the interpersonal level, but also within the context of social organisation and institutionalised techniques for social control. Foucault's works are also indicative of the limitations of any one discipline to accommodate the body while current notions of legitimate knowledge prevail, and much of the richness of his work comes from his disregard of normal disciplinary boundaries.

The work of Michel Foucault

Foucault argues for an understanding of the body which is essentially historical and located in the context of re-shaping the power of the state. In this process institutional mechanisms of social control, such as the prison, medical practice and the hospital focused attention on the body. In *Discipline and Punish* (1985a), *The Birth of the Clinic* (1976) and all three volumes of *The History of Sexuality* (1984c; 1986a; 1986b), Foucault argues, as did Elias (1978), that the body is the point of reference for processes of social control. Social control is about controlling the body. For Foucault, the body is controlled within a system of power/knowledge in which a discourse evolved to articulate the body. The development of discourse was a necessary condition for the power to control the body because power and knowledge are interdependent in Foucault's construction of social order. There can be no power to know without words, discourse, and articulation, which in turn function to constitute power. Such a constitution of power and discourse is relevant also to the construction of knowledges and discourse to the extent of being constitutive (or non-constitutive) of disciplines (branches of knowledge).

In *Discipline and Punish* (1985a) Foucault claims that the development of the prison system during the eighteenth and nineteenth centuries corresponded with a shift in conceptualising the body, a new discourse on the body, and changes in the relationship of the body to the state. The body was no longer the primary focus for punishment, as had been the case with public floggings, hangings and the like, being displaced by a more generalised form of punishment – imprisonment, which deprived the individual of liberty.

Accompanying this shift from the object body to the person's existential self was a move toward greater surveillance of the population in general, and especially within institutions. Power to control was integral with the power to know, and both required access to mechanisms of surveillance. One vehicle through which this surveillance was achieved, in prisons in particular, was the Panopticon, an architectural concept which allowed uninterrupted observation of inmates without their knowing they were being observed. In its typical form the Panopticon consisted of a central vantage point around which inmates' cells were located radially. It gained popularity as an architectural design for institutions like hospitals and prisons, and many examples of it still exist. As a design concept it is still regarded as a highly functional means of facilitating surveillance (although it is called 'observation') in hospitals, especially in intensive care units. Foucault saw it essentially as a means of maintaining power over people, structurally and socially.

It [the Panopticon] is a type of location of bodies in space, of distribution of individuals in relation to one another, of hierarchical organization, of disposition of centres and channels of power, of definition of the instruments and modes of intervention of power, which can be implemented in hospitals, workshops, schools, prisons (Foucault 1985a:205).

Not only did the Panopticon assist in the increasing surveillance of inmates, but it also evolved at a time when there was increasing surveillance of the population generally on the part of the state, particularly in public health and medicine. Foucault called this 'panopticism'. Hospitals, as institutions of the age of panopticism, made it possible for large numbers of people to be organised centrally and subjected to observation (surveillance) by medical practitioners. The hospital became an "examining" apparatus' at a time when medicine was beginning to make links between particular disease characteristics and demonstrable pathology, therefore establishing a rationale for the need to examine patients' bodies physically (Foucault 1985a:185). The body became the focus of attention as the causality of disease was transformed.

In *The Birth of the Clinic* (1976) Foucault traces the medicalisation of the object body, its reduction to a medical entity and the consequences of this for social order. He argues that there was an increasing emphasis on physical examination of both the living body and the corpse (in post mortem examinations) which allowed diseases to be identified and named. This development in medical practice not only facilitated evolution of a discourse about, and knowledge of, disease and pathology, it also brought power and state acceptance of the role of medicine in social order – a role which legitimised the 'medical gaze', that is, a way of looking at individuals that produced what Armstrong (1983) called a political anatomy of the body.

Nursing and surveillance of the body

Nurses also became concerned with surveillance (Foucault 1985a:186) in observing patients for changes in a range of bodily functions – a situation which endures to this day. The history of modern nursing is as much founded on observation of the patient as anything else. Florence Nightingale devoted more space to observation of the patient than to any other subject in *Notes on Nursing*, (first published in the 1850s) where she laid down her basic tenets of nursing. One of the most basic concepts that nurses are taught, which is taken for granted, and which goes unquestioned is 'observation makes the nurse'. As a principle of practice, observation is fundamental in contemporary nursing.

Nightingale also had a profound impact on hospital architecture. Leaving aside the emphasis she placed on fresh air and light which resulted in large windows and airy corridors (believed to minimise contagion emanating from foul air) in hospitals, the 'Nightingale ward' was a particular structure which allowed the nurse to observe all patients from one central location. The style was a rectangular adaptation of the radial Panopticon, but it allowed the same unbroken observation which panopticism demanded, and which the Panopticon provided.

In the post-Nightingale era, nurses became involved in widespread surveillance of the population through programs designed to improve child health. Nurses conducted large scale health screening and, through baby health clinics, they became heavily committed to monitoring mothering and child care practices. And they still emphasise the need to monitor and observe hospitalised patients.

The body, the state and AIDS

In very recent history, the AIDS epidemic has been associated with shifts in the way we conceptualise contagion (at least in the modern era), the body and its products, and we have witnessed what Cohen (1972) has described as a 'moral panic'.

Societies appear to be subject, every now and then, to periods of moral panic. A condition, episode, person or group of persons emerges to become defined as a threat to societal values and interests; its nature is presented in a stylised and stereotypical fashion by mass media; the moral barricades are manned [sic] by editors, bishops, politicians and other right-thinking people; socially accredited experts pronounce their diagnoses and solutions; ways of coping are evolved or (more often) resorted to; the condition then disappears, submerges or deteriorates and becomes more visible. Sometimes the object of the panic is quite novel and at other times it is something which has been in existence long enough, but suddenly appears in the limelight. Sometimes the panic passes over and is forgotten, except in folklore and collective memory; at other times it has more serious and long-lasting repercussions and might produce such changes as those in legal and social policy or even in the way society conceives itself (Cohen 1973:9).

In the AIDS epidemic we are seeing not only a moral panic but a paradigm shift (Kuhn 1970) in the way we think about the body. However, this particular shift reverts to more hysterical social responses to infectious disease, probably because the consequences of the disease are akin to previous great plagues, and so far science, which we have come to see as (almost) all powerful in such matters, has been unable to offer a cure. In the absence of a scientific solution, the social response is one which has been typical of previous great epidemics, however, this episode is compounded by moral issues which strike at the core of our value system, given that the stereotypical victims of the disease (homosexuals and intravenous drug users) are regarded as deviant. The state has a long history of intervention where moral issues are central to the debate, and under the guise of morality a range of social control measures, such as surveillance and custodianship, can be constructed as justifiable.

In the view put by Kroker and Kroker (1988b) the trend toward increasing surveillance which has been generated by the AIDS epidemic borders on panic such that in the United States 'hysteria over clean body fluids' and 'body McCarthyism' are justifying and legitimising greater surveillance of people, specifically their body fluids (Kroker & Kroker 1988b:10–12). In the 1980s AIDS bestowed new meaning to the body and it has created new symbolic dangers in things like blood and semen, and also possibly tears and saliva – products which were not previously regarded by westerners as inherently dangerous, at least not in a contagious sense.

The role of the state in surveillance of infected and potentially infected people has had a resurgence, and almost daily one hears debate about the relative merits of greater or lesser surveillance as a means to control the epidemic. Since AIDS was recognised as a major health problem we have witnessed a trend towards increasing surveillance that borders on panic (Kroker & Kroker 1988b).

In its relationship to the state, the body has a political presence to the extent that power to control the person is often mediated through the body. However, until the present decade this aspect of the body had been largely absent or silent in social theory and sociological work, as have other aspects of the body. The AIDS epidemic is having the effect of making the body more explicit as a social entity.

THE BODY IN SOCIAL THEORY

Berthelot succinctly summarised the place of the body in sociology in these terms:

> Although references to the body in the human and social sciences currently abound, a closer and more rigorous examination raises questions about their significance [such that] . . . sociology of the body [is] in such a state of dispersion, evanescence, precariousness and discontinuity that the original question of orientation has to be formulated: is there any meaning in a sociology of the body (Berthelot 1986:155)?

The disorganisation of the social science literature on the body illustrates the difficulty the body presents for sociologists, and Berthelot is sceptical of the current fashion to write the body into sociology. He argues that it has always been there both in reductive (1986:160) and scientifically acceptable guises such as diet, sexuality and beauty care (1986:155). He has suggested that we examine the body sociologically within a three level theoretical framework.

The first level involves viewing the body historically against a background of social movements. On this level the body could be studied in the context of social change, facilitating understandings of such things as the mechanisation of bodies at work during industrialisation (and the resultant 'mechanical man' notion). At the second level the body could be located sociologically within social thought, in particular within different ideologies which impact on the body. Thirdly, Berthelot argues for a level of analysis within the social sciences, that illustrates how psychology and psychoanalysis inscribe the body with a central role in social life (in psychopathology in particular). Additionally, ethnologists have accumulated a considerable cross cultural literature on the social body such that they (the social sciences) have constructed a 'complex social reality of the body' (Berthelot 1986:157). Berthelot's (1986:159) framework provides a useful conceptual schema for summarising a difficult area in sociology, particularly when one considers that

> the body is the particular site of an interface between a number of different domains: the biological and the social, the collective and the individual, that of structure and agent, cause and meaning, constraint and free-will. But this interface only emerges in sociological discourse because it is at the same time the objective centerpoint of the internal tension existing between the social and human science (sic: sciences) and because it is materialized in an irreducible, unique being: the

individual who is both object and subject, product and actor, structure and meaning.

However, although it is useful, Berthelot's three level approach still follows traditional sociological thinking and paradigms, all of which have so far failed to yield an adequate framework for the body in social life.

Creating space for the body

One of the most important recent attempts to address these theoretical problems is Turner's (1984) book, *The Body and Society: Explorations in Social Theory*. His central argument is that the body has not been taken seriously by sociologists, rather, they have 'desomatised' social relations (1984:231). He attributes the absence of the body to a 'theoretical prudery' resulting from sociology's attempts to dissociate itself from the biological determinism and positivism which characterised much nineteenth-century thought about human nature (Turner 1984:30–31). In effect, the rejection of biological determinism has resulted in what Turner (1984:31) calls 'sociological determinism', which has resulted in 'the exclusion of the body from the sociological imagination' because sociology had defined itself as a discipline concerned with the dichotomy of self/society, and not nature/culture.

Therefore, the development of sociology as a science of the 'purely' social, whatever that means, has not left a space for the body. The macro level, which concerns social structure, has no place for the body. The body is also excluded at the micro level where the focus is on the social construction of things, and Turner (1984:33) argues that any inclusion of the body at that level would raise the notion of individualism – that would be heretical.

Turner (1984:38–41) sets out what he believes to be the necessary elements of a sociology of the body. It must take account of body-self dialectic, that is, it must be interactive. It must distinguish between the individual self and that of populations, after Foucault's notion of the regulation of bodies in the regulation of populations. It must take account of the interface between biology and the social meanings imposed on that biology, in this sense it needs to be a political sociology. It must account for the inter-relationships between self and society, because 'the body is . . . crucial to both the micro and macro orders of society' (1984:40) and it must accommodate deviance and social control.

Added to these elements, Turner (1984:41) argues that a sociology of the body will be organised around four issues: 'reproduction and regulation of populations in time and space, and the restraint and the representation of body as a vehicle for the self'. Furthermore, it 'will hinge ultimately on the nature of the sexual and emotional division of labour' (1984:115) and a need to see the body's links to personhood and individual identity. Turner's view of a sociology of the body draws heavily on Foucault's work and on the belief that the body is intimately associated in human life with the need to control desire.

Like Berthelot (1986), however, Turner (1984) is still thinking in terms of existing disciplinary boundaries although he implies that if sociology is to theorise the body it must theorise the individual in order to accommodate body-self dialectic and to take account of a socially embodied self. Some authors have attempted to do that within an interactive social and economic framework (Featherstone 1982) and by a direct confrontation of the historical changes in ideas about nature, culture and the human body (Falk 1985). Feminists have made most progress to date, predominantly because feminist theory is critical of current modes of explanation and of disciplinary boundaries and because female embodiment has become a focal point for understanding women's experience.

Feminism, theory and the body

Many feminists have recently attempted to write the body into social life (Caddick 1986, Rothfield 1986, Haug 1987, Hite 1988, Grosz 1987, Gatens 1988, *Australian Feminist Studies* (5) 1987, Jaggar & Bordo 1989, Ussher 1989, Martin 1987). Most of this work is theoretical rather than empirical, with the exception of *Female Sexualisation* by Haug and others (1987), Ussher (1989) and Martin (1987), and it demonstrates the difficulty of existing disciplines and paradigms.

Caddick (1986) for example, illustrates an apparent absurdity in attempting to integrate the body and lived experience using existing epistemological and theoretical constructs. If one takes the body to be a biological given, one slips into the self/society paradigm and the body disappears, and 'just as the body exists as a theoretical absence, so it is projected as a vacant space in the actual interactions between persons in society' (Caddick 1986:67–68).

For women and feminists the body poses further difficulties because, as Rothfield (1986:158) explains, women are largely absent anyway, and 'to a degree, then, one confronts the following paradox or, rather, apparent contradiction: we are trying to theorise the body within a social and theoretical context which is structured (contingently) around its absence'. Rothfield (1986:165) goes further and argues that

> The wish to create a new space for the body requires more than pushing existing concepts together to make some room. Some radical revision is required. And this is the second point — there are some real difficulties for the attempt to write the body. On the one extreme reside the dangers of biologism and essentialism, and on the other, disembodiment. Somewhere in the middle, we hope, lies the body.

Although there is recognition of the need to re-think the body radically, no theory yet allows for the body in social life, but the task is a difficult one.

While the theoretical work is necessary, it is also the empirical work which is in urgent need of development; the problem, however, for empirical enquiry, has been finding a theoretical space in which to operate. Space for the body in sociology must take account of Turner's criteria, but it must also accommodate macro level analyses of the relationship of the body to production and reproduction, it cannot ignore feminist questions, and it must accommodate interpersonal social phenomena at the level of inter-group interaction. As well as all that, a theory of the body cannot ignore sexuality, because the human body in almost any social interaction is fundamentally a sexual and genderised entity. This is a daunting list for any discipline which is fundamentally concerned with social life and the body.

Space is being created by those who are examining the relationships between the body, sexuality, and social relations in a patriarchal society. Their work is discussed in the Chapter 3. We can also usefully look to anthropological work on the body and everyday social life, particularly that which concerns the social management of body products and their relationship to belief systems and taboos, and we can draw on analyses of the role of the body in culture.

NOTES

1. Personhood is an essentially human condition. It is state in which a self is constructed with and interacts with others and which is integrated and continuous with human physical form. Personhood is an experienced, given and acknowledged phenomenon that is to be understood in the context of bio-social interaction among humans. Personhood requires social life as well as physical life.
2. Although Martin Heidegger is acknowledged as having heavily influenced the

development of existentialism, including Sartre's work in this field, Heidegger's major publication on existential embodiment, *Being and Time*, was not translated into English until 1962, six years after Sartre's *Being and Nothingness* which was published in English in 1956 (see *Encyclopedia of Philosophy*, 1976, Volume 7, p.293, and Volume 3, p.464). Sartre's works also became well known beyond academic circles through his incorporation of existentialism into his major creative works. However, both Sartre and Heidegger draw substantially on the philosophical writings of Husserl, probably the most significant of all writers on existentialism.

3. Social life and the body

The body and social life interact in a number of ways. This chapter is about the interface between biology and culture and how it has been studied with respect to the body. There is only a small amount of literature on the subject, but it is important in illustrating that we cannot divorce culture and biology from each other.

THE BODY AND CULTURE

Cultural beliefs are linked to physical characteristics and both can be strong determinants of social life. There is an interdependent relationship between biology and culture that impacts on the body and is expressed bodily. For example, our patterns of social life would be vastly different if human women laid eggs and hatched them, or if men had babies – our parenting patterns and family relations would take account of different biological processes. Similarly, if the average woman was taller and physically stronger than the average man, relations among men and women would be different. The body is so basic to social life that Connell (1987: Ch. 4) has argued that it is the prime medium for interfacing the social and biological, and that it is via the body that biology is genderised.

Kern (1975) argues that the body is an important fundamental determinant of how we live our (social) lives. He demonstrates how potentialities for different life experiences are mediated by the object body and he points to aging, notions of beauty, physical size and other aspects of appearance to support his argument that the body is fundamental in structuring social relations. He says, for example, that 'a beautiful woman generally leads a vastly different life from a plain one' (1975:x). Even if one allows for such variable notions as what counts for beauty, he nevertheless points to how central the body is in social life. Physical appearance is both reflected

71

in, and a reflection of, social norms. Social life is experienced differently if one takes on, or has, a particular physical form. For example, a person of smaller than average height has a social life constructed in such a way that size is considered (see, for example, Walter De La Mare's *Memories of a Midget* and Ablon's 1984 study of dwarfs in the USA), taken for granted in social life and reflected in concepts such as 'the little man syndrome'. Similarly, if one is black, or has some obvious physical disfigurement (Goffman 1981) or dyes one's hair green, social relations will reflect difference from the norm. The body, however, can also be shaped by social norms, as was the case historically with the corset (Colmer 1979) and other practices which deform the body, such as Chinese foot binding, tattooing and the like (see Polhemus 1978:Part II A). It is, however, becoming increasingly difficult to identify just exactly what is now considered a 'normal' physical appearance in western culture, though there are discernable trends.

In contemporary society we are witnessing shifts in social norms towards more 'healthy' bodies, so that lifestyles are changing in pursuit of trimmer and fitter bodies. The body and parts thereof have different meanings in different cultures (and at different times within individual cultures) and this is especially critical, for example, in the case of a field researcher in a foreign land. Warren (1988:24–25) claims that

what is presented to the host culture is a body: a size and shape, hair and skin, clothing and movement, sexual invitation or untouchability. The embodied characteristics of the male and the female fieldworker affect not only the place in the social order to which he or she is assigned, but also the fieldworker's and informants' feelings about attractiveness and sexuality, body functions and display. Some of the way (sic:ways) in which the self is presented – such as hair style and clothing – can be altered; some – such as skin color and hand size – cannot.

Warren (1988:24–25) illustrates the integral and very practical relationships between culture and biology. However, attempts to address the body theoretically in relation to the interface between culture and biology have tended to be either predominantly social or biological. Some attempts have been made to explain cultural variations in the management of biological functions, however, they tend to return to biological determinism, as is the case with much psychoanalytic work, or they are descriptive only.

In western culture we tend to deal with the body by making it partly invisible and by constructing a series of rules to govern its exposure and its functions. The body is absent or silent in social theory and research, yet we nevertheless have taken-for-granted notions about how the body is to appear and be presented or controlled in our daily lives. We are an industrialised, clothed, and 'civilised' society but it has not always been that way.

THE CIVILISING PROCESS

One of the most significant works which addresses the management of the body in society, and one which forms part of the background to this study, is Elias' (1978) book, *The Civilising Process*. Elias describes a process which began around the eleventh century and produced a shift toward a more structured pattern of manners and a more prescriptive pattern of beliefs, norms and values about the body, body functions and body products. There was a major change in attitudes toward natural functions (1978:129) which became increasingly incorporated into beliefs about acceptable 'civilised' behaviour. The body was a major focus for this process so that it is possible to talk of a 'civilised' body.

The civilised body

As social norms about the body changed in response to the 'civilising process' the body has come to represent not only a thing in its own right, but also the source of processes and products which need control (civilising) or social management. According to Elias (1978:129–130), certain bodily functions such as farting and defaecating, which had previously been public acts, began to be privatised about the year 1530. Modesty in such matters was henceforth expected. For instance, in 1589 the Brunswick Court prescribed certain places for such bodily functions, and in 1619 Richard Westes published *The Booke of Demeanor and Allowance and Disallowance of Certain Misdemeanors in Companie*, which specified the need for modesty (privatising) of one's 'private parts' (Elias 1978:131–132).

Elias (1978:134) regards the increasing modesty over these bodily functions as a sign of civilisation, and he also notes that, from the 1600s, there was an increasing silence within writing explicitly dealing with body functions, especially during the middle 1700s. Furthermore, there was an increasing development of shame and embarrassment (which are not the same thing) as socially appropriate affective responses to some bodily functions (Elias 1978:135–136). The civilising process affects the way the body is managed in society, and there are consequences for sociology and nursing because, as Elias (1978:189–190) claims, the civilising process tends 'to make all bodily functions more intimate, to enclose them in particular enclaves, to put them "behind closed doors"', resulting in restraint over sexual matters and 'sociogenic shame and embarrassment'. In effect, the body becomes a thing to be controlled and many things associated with the body become taboo.

More and more, people keep the functions themselves, and all reminders of them, concealed from one another. Where this is not possible – as in marriage, for example – shame, embarrassment, fear, and all the other emotions associated with these driving forces of human life are mastered by a precisely regulated social ritual and by certain concealing formulas that preserve the standard of shame. In other words, with the advance of civilisation the lives of human beings are increasingly split between an intimate and a public sphere, between secret and public behaviour. And this split is taken so much for granted, becomes so compulsive a habit, that it is hardly perceived in consciousness (Elias 1978:190).

The civilising process has caused 'the gradual elaboration and internalisation (in the form of self-controls) of a whole series of taboos and precepts' which regulate body functions and exposure of the body (Waddington 1973:219). Taboos, which are not socially accepted topics for discourse, are also consequently not popular topics for research (see Faberow 1963:2).

Although the civilising process sounds feasible, there are a number of problems that Elias (1978) has not addressed. He writes about the process as though it is self-sustaining and he seems to imply that any culture which begins to 'civilise' will follow an apparently linear path toward increasing privatisation of a range of bodily functions. However, he offers no explanation about the mechanisms which sustain the process nor cause it to commence. Similarly, we have no way of knowing why excretion and sexuality, in particular, are singled out for a stricter form of privatisation than other functions such as blowing one's nose and eating. He has described a process which appears to end with what could be called 'Victorian' attitudes to the body and sexuality and does not take account of trends toward more openness with the body, sexuality and clothing which have developed over the twentieth century. The 'civilising process', for example, cannot explain the type of events which typified the 1960s, such as the Woodstock phenomenon, mini skirts and topless dresses, hippies and a return to more 'natural' lifestyles which have continued (if at rather uneven rates) into the present decade.

THE BODY AS A SYMBOL OF DIRT

Irrespective of the difficulties of the 'civilising process', we live in a society which proscribes certain acts in public, and we accommodate them architecturally and socially as private functions, especially excretion and sex. In this we are not alone, because it seems every culture has rules to govern certain acts, particularly those associated with dirt, and this includes some bodily functions (Douglas 1984).

The work of Mary Douglas

Mary Douglas' anthropological work on the social meaning and management of the body, which she outlined in her book, *Purity and Danger* (first published in 1966), has been extremely influential. Her central argument is that all cultures have symbolic systems which are fundamentally political and moral in nature, and which substantively concern pollution and dirt. The body is central in such systems because 'the body . . . provides a basic scheme for all symbolism. There is hardly any pollution which does not have some primary physiological reference' (1984:163–164). The functions and products of the body which she claims dominate symbolic systems are excretory or sexual – sometimes both. What is regarded as polluted (unclean or dirty) carries symbolic (and possibly real) dangers, but this is relative, because 'the difference between pollution behaviour in one part of the world and another is only a matter of detail' (1984:35).

For Douglas, therefore, there is a uniformity among cultures to the extent that human social systems establish ways of dealing with dirt, for example, avoidance, ritual, or sanctification, but there are differences between advanced and primitive societies.

One [difference] is that dirt avoidance for us is a matter of hygiene or aesthetics and is not related to our religion . . . [and] the second difference is that our idea of dirt is dominated by the knowledge of pathogenic organisms. The bacterial transmission of disease was a great nineteenth-century discovery. It produced the most radical revolution in the history of medicine. So much has it transformed our lives that it is difficult to think of dirt except in the context of pathogenicity. Yet obviously our ideas of dirt are not so recent. We must be able to make the effort to think back beyond the last 100 years and to analyse the bases of dirt-avoidance, before it was transformed by bacteriology; for example, before spitting deftly into a spitoon was counted unhygienic.

If we can abstract pathogenicity and hygiene from our notion of dirt, we are left with the old definition of dirt as matter out of place. This is a very suggestive approach. It implies two conditions: a set of ordered relations and a contravention of that order. Dirt then, is never a unique, isolated event. Where there is dirt there is system. Dirt is the by-product of a systematic ordering and classification of matter ... (Douglas 1984:35).

The body is the primary source of dirt, but such dirt is also imbued with a sense of power and sometimes danger, especially dirt associated with the margins of the body – excrement. All of this, however, has a cultural relativity such that, while all societies have some means of dealing with body dirt, there are characteristic belief patterns and practices within integrated symbolic systems and which typify particular cultures. Symbolic systems are, however, not fixed and Douglas argues that such systems are vulnerable at the margins where lines of demarcation are not as clearly defined.

All margins are dangerous. If they are pulled this way or that the shape of fundamental experience is altered. Any structure of ideas is vulnerable at its margins. We should expect the orifices of the body to symbolise its specially vulnerable points. Matter issuing from them is marginal stuff of the most obvious kind. Spittle, blood, milk, urine, faeces or tears by simply issuing forth have traversed the boundary of the body. So also have bodily parings, skin, nail, hair clippings and sweat. The mistake is to treat bodily margins in isolation from all other margins. There is no reason to assume any primacy for the individual's attitude to his [sic] own bodily and emotional experience, any more than for his cultural and social experience. This is the clue which explains the unevenness with which different aspects of the body are treated in the rituals of the world. In some, menstrual pollution is feared as a lethal danger; in others not at all .... . In some, death pollution is a daily preoccupation; in others not at all. In some, excreta is dangerous, in others it is only a joke (Douglas 1984:121).

Each culture, therefore, has its own pattern of beliefs about the dangers (or otherwise) of the body, body functions and body products, which reflect the pollution management processes and symbol systems of that culture. This is well illustrated in the Indian caste system where levels of contamination or pollution are associated with different castes. The lowest status in this system belongs to the so-called Untouchables, whose lives are governed not only by their low status, which they usually keep for life, but by roles associated with handling the dirt of those in higher castes. Various taboos and norms govern social relations among castes and the occupations they have, and can mean that some castes do not touch, look upon, or eat with those of another caste for fear of contamination. Douglas (1984:124) observed, for example, that touching excreta is particularly reviled in India so that people who clean toilets are amongst the lowest castes. It is possible, however, for lower castes to improve their status by emphasised adherence to rituals associated with pollution, and by taking on the behaviours of a higher caste (Worsley 1978:398).

Body products and excretion

Although anthropologists have studied rituals associated with the management of body products, especially excreta, they have ignored the actual body products (Loudon 1977). Furthermore, Loudon (1977:168) claims that 'as far as one can tell there are no human societies where the act of excretion and its products are not subject to public and private arrangements, to expectations involving time and space, regularity and appropriateness'. He also claims that in all societies buildings and areas are set aside for certain activities and that 'some such demarcations seem to apply to excretion; an important consideration in most cases seems to be the smell of human faeces' (1977:169). Loudon added a developmental factor, arguing that, during childhood, people learn to be either neutral or positive about their own excreta, but to have negative responses to the excreta of others. His explanation draws heavily on Freudian theory, investing certain body functions with psychological meaning, such as the ability of a child to exert control over others by producing or not producing excreta, particularly faeces. Loudon also emphasises smell because he says it is most influential in the vast majority of social mechanisms that have developed around body products.

Loudon's claims are consistent with those of Knapp (1967:587) who argues, again from a psychoanalytic perspective, that there is some innate need in humans to psychologically manage elimination and body products, and that there is an 'innate human tendency to shrink from objects which are slimy to the touch'. He goes so far as to claim that 'elimination processes play a part in more emotions than rage and disgust' (Knapp 1967:587). Although this work attempts to relate biology and social life, it essentially returns to biological determinism.

Much of the anthropological work on the body has been influenced by a psychoanalytic perspective with an underlying biological determinism. It is therefore important to examine a small area of the psychoanalytic literature on the body and body products which began with a paper by Kubie in 1937. He explicitly argues for an innate human approach to body products.

THE KUBIE HIERARCHY OF DIRT

Kubie (1937:388) proposed that, while the individual had no in-nate sense of 'dirt', people developed an 'emotional judgement' about dirtiness and cleanness as a result of experience of the ego with the environment. Such experiences, he claimed, lead to un-conscious fantasies about dirt, and these fantasies – many of them to do with the genitalia – affect the way people behave in their social lives. He added that (western) people are confused about dirt, having many ideas which were contradictory, paradoxical and absurd (1937:389). He claims that there are some consistencies about the ways humans dealt with the body, for example, that humans do not use, as food, animal tissue associated with apertures or what issues from them – in effect, what is considered dirt. Such observations would seem to be selective, or culturally relative, given that some delicacies are made from just those parts of the body Kubie said we did not eat, such as pigs' heads (used to make brawn), eyes, testicles, the parson's nose of poultry, tripe and other intestines.

The body, for Kubie (1937:391) is a 'dirt factory' and he sub-scribes to a psychological definition of dirt as 'anything which either symbolically or in reality emerges from the body, or which has been sullied by contact with a body aperture'.

As part of his psychological explanation of dirt, Kubie proposed a 'tacit hierarchy of dirt', embedded in the unconscious. In his schema, the hierarchy is organised on a dimension of cleanness and dirtiness, with tears probably being considered the cleanest, and faeces and urine falling near the bottom. He did not propose a place in this arrangement for two products, milk and semen, because he said people would have 'the most perplexing ambivalence' (1937:395) about them, although he did not say why this should be the case. To order his hierarchy further, he proposed four assump-tions which he said were encountered 'almost universally' in fantasy.

(1) Softness, wetness, sliminess, and hairiness, respectively, are always looked upon as dirtier than hardness, dryness, and the absence of hair. (2) Old age represents a piling up of undischarged remnants of a lifetime of eating and drinking, and is dirtier than youth. So that growing old means to grow dirty; and infants, although in the unconscious they may be made from faeces, are nevertheless and paradoxically cleaner than age. (3) Furthermore, pigmentation obviously means dirt, and dark hair is dirtier than the blond hair which 'gentlemen prefer'. And (4) finally in general a prominent or out-jutting part of the body carries a presumption of cleanliness, whereas a cavity,

or cleft, or hole, or pit in the body carries the presumption of dirt (Kubie 1937:395).

Kubie also proposed that smooth skin would be considered cleaner than skin which was wrinkled, as it is on the penis and scrotum, and that thin people would be perceived as cleaner than fat ones, but 'the most important single consequence of this hierarchy of fantasies ... [is] an unconscious but universal conviction that woman is dirtier than man' (1937:396). Added to this is a taboo associated with the apertures such that 'by every means, and by varying degrees at different times and in different civilisations, the apertures have been camouflaged' (1937:396).

To develop his theory, Kubie selectively used data from ethnographic and anthropological studies as well as observations from his practise as a psychoanalyst. Leach (1958) is extremely critical of the inappropriate and at times inaccurate use of anthropological studies to support psychoanalytic explanations of human behaviour. He argues that anthropological concepts are taken out of context and invested with psychological meaning – meaning which, in many cases, is contextually and culturally specific. Although Leach's comments were made with particular reference to the work of another psychoanalyst, his criticisms could equally apply to Kubie. In effect, Kubie was using socially derived data to support an essentially biological construction of human behaviour.

Kubie's hypotheses abound with serious flaws, debatable assumptions, and multiple biases, not the least of which is sexism. However, three decades later his work provoked a spate of empirical studies, again within psychoanalytic traditions (Ross et al 1968, Kurtz et al 1968, Hirt et al 1969, Dimond & Hirt, 1974) which are intriguing. In each study the authors claimed to have demonstrated support for the Kubie hierarchy.

Ross et al (1968) tested Kubie's model using a 7 point semantic differential scale. They were interested in demonstrating the existence or non-existence of a clean-dirty dimension of 21 body products[1] deduced from Kubie's proposal. In an initial exploratory study they tested two groups of medical students, and a smaller group of nursing and social work students. Acknowledging that these groups were not representative of the population in general they tested a larger sample consisting of '203 white males, 59 white females, and 11 Negroes (mostly male)' (1968:305). The age of the sample was skewed towards the 20–30 years group, but the sample was judged to be reasonably representative. The results showed a high level of consistency among the people studied, such that, for each of the 21 body products, there was little variation in the rank ordering of products according to their perceived cleanness or dirtiness. Tears, which Kubie had suggested would be considered clean, were indeed rated among the cleanest, and those products which he hypothesised would rate as dirty, were judged that way. The two products (milk and semen) about which Kubie suggested there would be ambivalence were rated among the cleanest of body products. The only product where there was a rating inconsistency between the groups concerned the medical students who rated faeces 'more dirty' than did the other two groups. The authors concluded that their research showed 'considerable confirmation for Kubie's description of a 'hierarchy of the products of the body'' (1968:308).

However, the authors do not say whether or not the participants in their study were asked to answer in terms of their own body products, or those of other people, though, from the results they published, one suspects the subjects rated other people's body products. This seems a remarkable oversight given that Kubie theorised that people make positive/negative differentiations on the basis of self and other. Also, there is a reported differential rating of faeces by medical students, relative to the other groups, and yet the authors make no comment about the possible causes of the difference other than to say that there was the possibility it might reflect the 'psychological or subcultural characteristics' (1968:307–308) of the group. Neither do the authors say whether the difference is statistically significant. The authors also report, without either explanation or analysis, that 'not surprisingly, . . . [menstrual blood] is . . . ranked eighth from the 'clean end' of the order by women, whereas it is ranked thirteenth (or ninth from the 'dirty end') by the men' (1968:307). (The subject of women's bodies, including menstruation, is discussed in Chapter 4.)

A second study, by Kurtz et al (1968), reports similar data. Again results are in the form of reported responses on a 7 point semantic differential scale, to 20 of the same 21 body products used by Ross and others (nail clippings were omitted), but this time dimensions of evaluation, potency and activity replaced dirtiness/cleanness. The sample consisted of: two groups of medical students (N=22 per group); 10 female graduate nursing students; and 10 female social work students. Factor analysis of the subjects' ratings of the 20 body products suggested a single factor could account for 70–80% of the total variance. There were no remarkable differences among or between groups, nor between the sexes, and again there was a consistent hierarchy of affective responses to body products. In this study there is the implication that subjects could have been asked for responses to their own body products, rather than those of another person but, like the Ross et al (1968) study, that is not made clear. The same rank ordering of products appears – tears and human milk were among the 'cleanest', while pus and blackheads were among the 'dirtiest'. In these samples there was a consistent tendency for all products to be rated towards the 'dirty' end of the scale, reflecting a generalised negative affective response to body products.

The third study, by Hirt et al (1969) used the same 21 products that Ross et al (1968) had used, and again there was a 7 point semantic differential scale with dimensions of evaluation, potency, and activity. They used a sample of 205 adults described as 'unselected job applicants at a large factory' (1969:486) who ranged in age from 20–62 years, with schooling and socio-economic backgrounds representing a cross-section of the community. The sample was divided by sex, class (high, middle, and low socio-economic status) and age (<30 and >30 years) and the researchers found no significant differences between the groups. Rather, they found, as the other two groups of researchers did, a very high level of consistency in the rating of all 21 body products. Again milk and tears were the highest scorers, and pus and blackheads were the lowest rated products. Again subjects used the low end of the scale, indicating to the researchers that there was a generalised negative attitude to most body products. The authors concluded that 'the major finding . . . [was the existence of] a consistent hierarchy of attitudes toward body products' (1969:489) which they said Kubie had accurately anticipated. On the meaning of such a hierarchy the authors were uncertain.

Dimond and Hirt (1974) used the same approach as the three studies reported above, but in their study, Dimond and Hirt tested hospitalised schizophrenics (N=25), hospitalised paraplegics (N=25), and 'normals' who were 'volunteers solicited from a local businessmen's club' (1974:251)(N=25). Using a 7 point scale for the same 21 products, they analysed responses to 9 bi-polar adjectives. Using factor analysis, they found, unlike Kurtz et al. (1968), that they could not account for most of the variance on one factor alone.

However, they did find the same highly consistent hierarchical ordering of responses to body products among all three groups.

They remarked that this was most noteworthy for schizophrenics who tend to differ from non-schizophrenics on 'virtually every task examined' (1974:252) with the exception of their responses to body products. They concluded, as did the other three groups of researchers, that the Kubie model is not only supported by their research, in both the pattern and intensity of results, but also that there was the same high level of consistency.

THE MEANING OF DIRT AND THE BODY

What all this research on dirt and the body might mean, of course, is another matter. While Kubie started from a Freudian point of view, and while there are many limitations to that view, it does not detract from the evidence, which suggests a consistent and highly reproducible pattern of responses to body products, at least for some cultural groups. All of the studies mentioned were conducted in North America, so the results may only be indicative of cultural patterns in that part of the world, and in closely related cultures. The consistency of the results, however, is persuasive. These studies have some relevance for a sociological analysis of the ways nurses manage the body, but one added complication for nurses, is that they are required to deal with a range of situations where body products could not be said to be 'normal'.

The beliefs and motivations behind the Kubie pattern, and the hierarchical ordering of the body products requires further work, which goes beyond the scope of my study. It is fair to say, though, that the literature support the notion that all societies have ways of dealing with the body, body products and dirt – irrespective of how it is defined. It also seems clear that there is a very close nexus between the body, sexuality and dirt, and the social mechanisms which govern and proscribe behaviour related to them. It also seems clear that within any culture there are patterns of beliefs which are explored and elaborated to regulate the body. In our society, there is the notion of the 'civilising process' which locates our particular ways of dealing with the body, sexuality and dirt within a privatising context, rendering them relatively inaccessible to us as a subject of social enquiry. Consequently we do not have to be explicit about such matters unless normal social order is disrupted. Alternatively, we can turn to psychoanalytic explanations about our bodies, but that too absolves us from a sense of responsibility to know and understand them – if they are related to unconscious and innate urges, then we have no need to understand them socially.

My aim is to document how one group of nurses manages the bodies of other people, not only in performing physical care, but also how they manage the body products of others.

Nurses have a degree of access to bodies and a need to know about the body that is incomparable to any other group. This not only presents them with difficulties, but it also means that if any group in our society knows (experientially and practically) about the body, nurses do.

Studies of the various body products have demonstrated a consistent tendency for body products to induce a negative affect, and there is no evidence to suggest this is not so for Australians. Therefore, I was interested to explore the methods nurses, who work directly with body products and bodies, use to manage their reactions in their normal work. To date there is little literature, beyond that which concerns dirty work, that one can turn to for the development of a social analysis of the body and body products, and there is little empirical literature about the body in either the social sciences or nursing. There are, however, some clear theoretical guidelines that can facilitate empirical work, particularly with respect to documenting the ways in which the body and body products are managed in this culture. In the first instance, it is necessary to identify what beliefs and practices govern the body and what we take for granted about its exposure, its sexuality, and its relationships to other aspects of our belief system. In part, that is what I wanted to explore in this study.

NOTE
1. The 21 body products were: ear wax, desquamated cells between the toes, nose pickings, hair, faeces, semen, human milk, dandruff, face sweat, saliva, blood, vomit, menstrual discharge, blackheads, tears, pus, phlegm, nail clippings, pubic hair, body sweat and urine.

4. The body and sexuality

In becoming 'civilised' (Elias 1978) sexual aspects of life have become privatised. However, unlike other privatised bodily functions such as excretion and bathing, sexual behaviour (acts defined as sexual) and sexuality (the experience of and others' perceptions of people as sexual beings) are social constructions which are built around the biological differences between the male and female body. Sexual aspects of social life are considerably more complex than is the case for other features of embodied existence because: (1) they are integral both to the meanings associated with gendered and sexualised behaviour, and to relations between men and women; and (2) sexuality and sexual behaviour are products of the interrelation of biology and culture.

This means that bodies, body products and sexuality never come without a great deal of cultural 'baggage' so that, when nurses are confronted with a particular patient, cultural meanings which attend being either a nurse or a patient and the context of care all require management. Much of that management concerns the meanings attached to: (1) the biological body and its functions; (2) the definitions that patients and nurses place on the relationship between the physical body and sexual expression; (3) the experience of embodiment; and (4) experiences of touching the bodies of others and being touched.

Given the nature of sexuality and sexual behaviour in our culture, it is not surprising that by far the most problematic areas of the body for the nurse (and probably also for the patient) are those associated with sexuality and genitalia. For several reasons this is especially so where male patients are concerned. Firstly, most nurses are females, and the nurse-patient encounter is a social event where gender needs to be managed. Secondly, masculinity and the power of males over females is enacted through the body and it centres on the penis. Thirdly, nursing activities often require

85

a level of intimacy not usually experienced outside sexual contexts. Fourthly, nurses experience sexual harassment from male patients as women do elsewhere in society, however, nurses face the added problem of sometimes having to continue on-going physical and nursing care for the harasser.

Ours is a patriarchal society, and this is clearly illustrated in the genderised social meanings of the body, sexuality and sexual behaviour. We have one sexuality for women, and another for men – it is not a case of sex-specific variations of the same theme. Sexuality, as against physical sexual characteristics, is not biologically given, though it is often conceptualised that way by those who have studied it within the dominant logic-positivist and dualistic approach. However, 'the fact that women can bear children and men cannot has influenced the way in which female and male sexuality is conceptualised and regulated in most cultures' (Warren 1986:142). The meaning and expression of sexual being are inextricably located in the (believed) biologically given nature and functions of the external genitalia (and in the internal genitalia of women) and their social meanings and symbolism.

Sexuality, when it has been the subject of enquiry, has almost always been epistemologically fragmented, as have other aspects of embodied existence. Many studies (probably most) and much of the theoretical work have been conducted from perspectives which support dominant world views, especially with respect to genetically based sex differences (Rogers 1988). The psychoanalytic approach, which originated outside a dominant perspective but which came to be extremely influential, also relies heavily on biological determinism. With the exception of (most) feminism, sexuality has been conceptualised as a biological given in which social processes play a greater or lesser, though secondary, part.

SEXUALITY AND WESTERN CULTURE

As a subject of empirical social enquiry, sexuality has not had a high profile in western culture (Bullough 1972) and what exists has masculine bias (Gunew 1987). Bullough (1972) claims that sexuality, and associated phenomena such as courtship, have been avoided by historians, and that what histories of sexuality have been written tend to have a sense of moral disapproval. For example, homosexuality, when it has been the subject of enquiry by historians, has been discussed in disapproving terms, though other disciplines such as psychology, anthropology and sociology, have not usually been so morally judgmental, or at least not explicitly so.

Padgug (1979) argues that there has been no single thematic approach to the historical analysis of sexuality, rather, there is a tendency to see sexuality from a contemporary viewpoint, and this results in a construct of sexuality which is ahistorical. He argues that an adequate discussion of sexuality is difficult because sexuality is an interface between the public and the private, and because it also has political and economic implications in the sense that sexuality and production interrelate. Padgug also emphasises that, although sexuality is a combination of the social and the biological, human sexuality is heavily influenced by social learning. Becoming human requires social interaction but we cannot simply 'peel off' the social to reveal the underlying biology (Padgug 1979:10). This is particularly so of sexuality, he claims, and therefore, an adequate analysis of human sexuality requires integration of the social with the biological, as the earlier discussion of the nature of the body established.

In 1982, Vincinus reviewed the literature on sexuality and observed that it was a field where the authors were mostly white males and that, in general, the subject had been treated in one of three ways: lost and submerged histories of marginal groups (gay men, lesbians, prostitutes); histories of ideas and social movements; and social structures of sexuality – behaviours, definitions, and politics. It was a literature which she described as heavily oriented toward 'boundary-keeping', that is, deciding what is normal or deviant (Vincinus 1982:135), and biased in favour of a heterosexual male model of sexuality. This heterosexual male model emphasises the energy-control or hydraulic model of sexuality centred on the male orgasm.

Sexuality and sexually expressive behaviour have generally been conceptualised as androcentric, phallocentric, essentially copulatory in nature, and heterosexuality is taken to be the norm. This is not only a consequence of a patriarchal society, but also a function of a construction of knowledges which reflects the reality of the dominant group – white men of relatively high status. With respect to nurses' practice, this relationship of sexuality and sexual behaviour to patriarchy presents particular difficulties when the patient is male and his (sexualised) body is a source of vulnerability, if not physical weakness, and he must rely on a woman for help.

Sexuality and sexual behaviour are also a part of social life where the male role is defined as dominant and proactive, while the female role is defined as passive and receptive. Berg (1986:165–166) observes that

> there is a strong tendency in our culture for sexual interaction to be viewed as something that is properly done by men to women. 'He screwed her' is in common usage; 'she fucked him' is not. Presumably this reflects the way in which Australian men are generally encouraged from an early age to behave in an active and dominant manner in relation to women, while Australian women are generally encouraged to be passive and submissive in relation to men.

What Berg describes should not be seen as only a problem of structuring roles in sexual encounters, it is also quite basically a problem of language (symbolism) – a language which reflects a particular construction of reality in sexual matters.

Language and sexuality

The *Macquarie Dictionary* (1985), a standard reference for the Australian usage of English, defines sexuality as a noun, meaning: '1. sexual character; possession of sex. 2. the recognition or emphasising of sexual matters'. Such a definition, while not very helpful when phrased in those terms, becomes more meaningful when the entry for the adjective 'sexual' is examined:

> 1. of or pertaining to sex. 2. occurring between or involving the two sexes. 3. having sex or sexual organs, or reproducing by processes involving both sexes, as animals or plants. 4. having a strong sex drive or having the ability to arouse strong sexual interest.

The primary notion in these definitions is that sex is a biological construct. The entry for sexual intercourse, however, is a very clear illustration of the heterosexual, male-oriented, copulatory and biologico-dominant model of sexuality which prevails. Sexual intercourse, a noun, is said to be: 'the insertion of the penis into the vagina followed by ejaculation; coitus; copulation'.

Ruth (1987), writing from a North American perspective, claims that the language of sexuality betrays an ambivalence and hysteria about sexuality in western patriarchy. She says that when language is used at all to describe copulation it is sexist, and usually slang. There is no expressive, explanatory term to describe it other than mechanical copulatory words (Ruth 1987:151). She explains it in these terms:

> One may have sex, have sex with, copulate with, make love to, lie with, sleep with, take someone to bed (none of these terms even near

accurate representations), but one cannot simply —— (insert appropriate verb). In the slang one can simply ——, yet for nonsexist people the slang will not work. Were it even less illicit, less associated with and connotive of the sleazy, the current slang lexicon would still be inadequate to capture the range of activities and experiences involved. Essentially masculist, its terms are single-mindedly genital and almost exclusively heterosexual. What is more, they are violent and contemptuous, sharply reflective of the society and the mind-set that give rise to them.

How odd that this ubiquitous animal activity claims in our language no acceptable verb that expresses precisely what one does when one does it! To sex? To sex someone or sex oneself or be sexed. Sexing, the act of. In the absence of anything better, this term will have to do.

It seems, at first, peculiar that we should be in such a quandry to find a word for an event so common in human experience. Generally, language reflects society's reality (Ruth 1987:151).

Ruth (1987:153–154) goes on to argue that in the absence of 'polite' language to describe 'sexing' we have little choice other than to use words commonly regarded as 'foul' or 'dirty' and that 'we are taught, when one mucks about with sex/sexuality in our culture, one lowers oneself to the dirt'. Furthermore, 'the foul repertoire reveals that the worst of our terms or epithets [about sexing] refer to body parts and functions' (Ruth 1987:154).

In language, therefore, sexuality shares a space similar to some aspects of the privatised body – secreted away and talked of in terms which are either sanitised or regarded as vulgar. Sexuality, sexual expression and sexual behaviour are beyond the margins of acceptable social discourse. Alternatively, sexuality is reduced to biology and talked of with language and concepts associated with disciplines such as biology and physiology. Acts of 'sexing' – to take a term from Ruth (1987) – can therefore be dealt with in a way which excludes social, experiential and personal knowledge.

There is another aspect to the language of sexuality which locates sexuality within the context of power differences between men and women. Hartsock (1984) argues, for example, that words (which also therefore represent our particular constructs of sexuality) such as 'bang' or 'screw' reveal power and violence in sexual language. Germaine Greer (1971:41) also noted this linguistic phenomenon and she claimed that 'all the linguistic emphasis is placed upon the *poking* element; *fucking, screwing, rooting, shagging*, are all performed upon the passive female: the names for the penis are all *tool* names'.

If it is true, as Ruth (1987:154) suggests, that 'sex-talk is a map of sex-thought', western culture has its contradictions about sexuality.

In patriarchy sex-thought is decidedly schizophrenic: sexing exists, and it does not exist. *For the record* it is absent, what one might call a non-event, something which happens which yet does not happen. Too disturbing, too out of sync with the patriarchal construction of life, too dissociating even to utter, sexuality is ,unspeakable', not formally acknowledged, and so in 'official' public awareness it is erased, in a sense deactualized. It is reactualized only in different, even quarantined, psychic locations: either in the medico-technical retreat, where it may be isolated, scrubbed of affect, and rendered harmless, or in the nether regions of some sleazy, subordinate reality, where slang and id and sin reside (Ruth 1987:154).

In effect, sexuality does not fit into socially acceptable language, our social world or our configuration of knowledges. As an aspect of being, the concept of 'sexuality' shares similar problems to the concept of 'body' because understanding these notions theoretically requires a more integrative framework than that which is in general usage. Notions of the body and sexuality must be understood in the context of what they symbolise within a system of beliefs and social practices. However, there is the added problem of their marginal status as topics of legitimate investigation or discourse and as topics which overlap moral and religious issues. In Mary Douglas' (1984) view, sexuality and some aspects of the body, particularly physiological processes, lie on the margins of what is considered dangerous and potentially polluting and as such they are subjected to social management and control.

The need to control the body

The reason for the linguistic and social difficulties with sexuality and the body, for western culture, is said by some to lie in our Judaeo-Christian heritage (Featherstone 1982, Turner, 1982, 1984, Foucault 1984c, 1985a, 1985b, 1986a, 1986b, Aries 1985), which emphasised the need to control the body as it came to be regarded as the source of sinful urges and desires. There is a strong religious link between the body, sexual behaviour, sexuality and sinfulness. Foucault's work in this area has been highly influential, particularly to the extent that he was able to trace historical links between disciplinary practices and institutions, and concepts of the body as a thing to be controlled by both the state and the individual. Foucault's work has also been comprehensively incorporated into current thinking on sexuality, but he is not without his critics.

Weeks (1981:8–10) argues that Foucault has not added much to the work in this area, rather it simply appears this way because the

French have been intellectually provincial in their use of the literature and history, and furthermore, that sexuality is not a given to be controlled as Foucault suggests, but an 'historical construct that has historical conditions of existence' (Weeks 1981:10). Lynch (1987:143–144) claims that, among other things, Foucault does not take account of gender in his discussions of the body nor does he consider corporeality (sexuality) as it is experienced. Keat (1986:30–31), however, argues that Foucault's discussion of the repression of sexuality is tied too closely to a psychoanalytic model (which is itself a form of discourse/power) and that there is a hidden 'naturalism' (biologism) in Foucault's notion of human nature because he sees humans as primarily motivated by pleasure and leisure.

In the Judaeo-Christian tradition, the body became a 'bad' thing and its sexual urges particularly bad, leading to so-called 'sins of the flesh' or 'sins against the body'. Aries (1985:37) argues that some sexual practices which were primarily used to enhance pleasure were rendered sinful in the translation of some texts from their original Latin. Such sins, he says, which were called 'sins against the body' could constitute one of the great inventions of Christian religion.

Explaining and scientising sexuality

Religion provides a way of understanding the world, and this includes an understanding of the body and sexuality. Christianity has promoted the body as a thing which needs control, especially with respect to sexuality, sexual behaviour and sexual expression. In such a framework, being a good Christian means gaining control of the body and its sexual urges. Conceptually this is an uncomplicated way of understanding the body and sexual being, however, as science has progressively replaced religion as a source of knowledge about the world, explanations have become more elaborate and emphasis on empiricism means that some topics are accommodated better than others. For instance, death (as a subject, and as a subject related to the body) does not lend itself to empirical enquiry (although dying does) and it has been largely ignored by academia. However, sexuality and sexual behaviour have been subjected to enquiry, but as topics of research, they have remained on the fringes of legitimacy. This is more the case for sexuality than for sexual behaviour because the latter has been studied, for example, by Masters and Johnson (1966). Despite the rigor of their research or the importance of their ideas, those who have studied sexuality and sexual behaviour have been regarded with suspicion and scepticism, especially if they operated outside established paradigms and theories, for example, Kinsey et al (1949, 1953), Freud (1965, 1979a, 1979b) and Hite (1976).

One of the best known of all writers on matters of a sexual nature was Freud whose many theories of human development, personality, and psychopathology, are pervaded by notions of the need of the psyche to constantly battle with the body and sexual urges. Freud's view, which came to be so influential, was that the body was an essentially sexual entity, and the psyche – the controlling centre for personality – was primarily concerned with integration of innate and biologically determined sexual urges into socially accepted behaviours.

To those who followed Freud, and Freud himself, human nature was essentially sexual, and there was a sexual metaphor in seemingly all aspects of life. Bejin (1985:181) claims that 'Freud discovered "sexuality" . . . and invented the science of sex', although there had been earlier works on the subject published in the mid 1800s, the most famous of which is *Psychopathia Sexualis*, published firstly by Heinrich Kaan and secondly by Krafft-Ebing. Freud began a process which saw an increasing scientising and psychologising of sexuality, but much of his work, such as his notions of repression, transference and the unconscious is inaccessible to science. In many ways, his ideas are incompatible with a scientised understanding of sexuality but they have been particularly enduring.

In 1922 Wilhelm Reich, whose work is closely related to that of Freud, discovered what he termed 'orgasmic power', and in 1942 he published *The Function of the Orgasm* (1975). He emphasised the hydraulic model of human physiology which was popular at the time, but Reich's thesis was truly radical to the extent that he believed that regular orgasm was absolutely fundamental to good health. He raised sexuality, as it were, to a therapeutic plane and made the orgasm central in his theory of good health.

According to Jackson (1984a) Havelock Ellis' work was also highly influential in providing a 'scientific' rationale and 'evidence' which condoned differential experiences of men and women in sexual relations. Prevailing attitudes to male sexuality were largely confirmed by Ellis' writings, although he did emphasise the need for women to experience sexual pleasure. His work was Darwinian and 'naturalistic' and did not question the taken-for-granted notions of 'normal' sexual expression. Rather, Jackson (1984a) argues that the work of Ellis is an illustration of how science legitimised male dominance and the male's 'need' for sexual gratification – a 'need' believed to be biologically determined. This notion about male sexuality has also been particularly enduring.

In the 1940s and 1950s, Kinsey and others (1948, 1953) studied sexual experiences using behaviouristic and physiological methodologies which were popular at the time. To Kinsey and his fellow researchers, sexual experience was reduced to a series of categories such as frequency of intercourse and choice of partners. Bejin (1985:183) argues that Kinsey's work generated a mode of analysis which placed the orgasm at the centre, rendering other aspects of sexual experience peripheral. He claims that these studies were not sexology, but 'orgasmology' whereby sexual therapy became 'orgasmotherapy'. In Kern's (1975:138) view, Kinsey's work rendered sexuality 'a competitive event subject to the same kinds of evaluations on the basis of speed, frequency, and endurance previously reserved for athletic events and machine production'.

The scientising of sexual behaviour progressed further with Masters and Johnson's book, *Human Sexual Response*, in 1966. This work gave detailed accounts of the physiological and behavioural responses to sexual arousal and orgasm. Normal sexual function was defined in terms of being orgasmic, and sexual dysfunction amounted to being anorgasmic. In this sense, therefore, scientised sexuality was constructed as mechanical, copulatory, and physiological, with little attention being given to affective, existential (experiential) or social phenomena. To Masters and Johnson (1966) there was little place for what I have called sexuality, rather, their work is concerned with sexual behaviour – it is primarily physiological, biological, reductive and positivist. Again the orgasm is the centrepiece of sexual experience and to them sexuality and sexual behaviour are the same thing – a set of observable phenomena.

Positivist studies like those of Masters and Johnson (1966) decontextualise sexual experiences. Kupfermann (1979:16–19) is highly critical of such methods of studying sexual experience and sexual expression and argues that they are characteristic of our mechanistic and technological age and a 'tinkering' mentality. She not only claims that the highly successful but controversial Hite Report (1976) epitomises this approach by separating the body from the psyche. She says that in Hite's analysis 'the toolshop is never far away in such concepts as "adequate lubrication", and "genital stimulation"' (Kupfermann 1979:18). Kupfermann's most serious criticism, however, is reserved for Masters and Johnson whom she claims deny the experiential component of sexuality, that is, they emphasise the body and its biology in sexual physiology and ignore the rich social meanings which accompany human sexuality (Kupfermann 1979:19). For Kupfermann, and many others, especially women, sexuality is part of being. Sexualising and genderising are integral to the development of a personal identity – a process which cannot be reduced to a set of physiological responses.

Kupfermann explains what she means by this, and her experiences place her in a unique position to illustrate the extent to which the body is culturally symbolic.

In my teens, as an aspiring starlet and model, I was initiated into the sacred world of the 'beauty-culture', and I observed my body almost objectively in a detached fashion, as it was moulded into an object of glamour. I was daily pummelled, pushed, tonged and tweezed, and certainly by today's liberated standards I was a sex-object, a dolly, who, passive, allowed herself to be primed and painted like a blank canvas every day by a team of technicians. At this point my only 'body awareness' was of my body's boundary; of shape and line, of light and shade; of creating magical auras with hair and gloss . . . .
In my twenties, when I became a mother, I discovered another dimension to my body – its inner spaces, and biological rhythms. This is not to say I was totally unaware of them before, but pregnancy and childbirth has a way of dramatically and often rudely focusing one's attention to these inner voices: it forces every woman to confront her body in the raw, as it were – and certainly the handling many women receive during childbirth brings a sharp awareness, perhaps for the first time, of the body as a 'lump of meat', and of animal affinities (Kupfermann 1979:10–11).

It is in the area of women's bodies – becoming sexualised, or depersonalised and reduced to bodies – that much of the more recent work on the body and sexuality is being done, mostly by women, and mostly within feminist traditions. Such work provides a perspective from which to view the existential aspects of embodiment, and the symbolic meanings attached to women's bodies and men's bodies, and it also provides a framework for analysing social and sexual relations between and among men and women. Men are also beginning to explore the relationships between the body (especially the genitalia), sexuality, and masculinity, but to date they have not moved as far into existential or empirical frameworks as much as feminist writers have.

MEN'S BODIES, SEXUALITY AND MASCULINITY

The male body and genitalia are inextricably interrelated with the meanings and expression of masculinity and sexuality. In male sexuality the penis is paramount, and within patriarchal society the penis is the single most important anatomical symbol which represents masculinity. Compared with female sexuality, male sexuality is more genital, less diffuse and more concerned with power and performance and it is more physical.

Weeks (1981:39) argues that the contemporary interrelationship of anatomy and symbol in male sexuality and sexual behaviour began around the 1830s when handbooks on manhood started to appear. Beliefs linking sexuality, masculinity and power, which these texts promoted, were also supported through major social developments such as sport, schools (especially private schools), male clubs, and militarism. The nexus between male sexuality, masculinity and power became institutionalised within a patriarchal system. The consequences of this process for men are only now being recognised within sociology (Connell 1983, Metcalf & Humphries 1985, Brod 1987), but the consequences for both men and women have long been recognised by feminists. Very little, however, has been written on the subject of male bodies, in contrast to that which exists on female bodies (see, for example, Strang 1984, Warner 1985), particularly as it relates to imagery of women's bodies in pornographic and erotic media. Masculinity and male sexuality have also been little studied, either theoretically or empirically.

Connell (1983, 1987), who is one of the few to have studied masculinity, links masculinity not only to sexuality and the physical body, but he also integrates social action and meaning. He says of maleness that it is

not a simple thing. It involves size and shape, habits of posture and movement, particular physical skills and the lack of others, the image of one's own body, the way it is presented to other people and the ways they respond to it, the way it operates at work and in sexual relations. In no sense is all this a consequence of XY chromosomes, or even of the possession on which discussions of masculinity have so lovingly dwelt, the penis. The physical sense of maleness grows through a personal history of social practice, a life-history-in-society (Connell 1987:84).

For Connell, masculinity in western society is predominantly learned through institutionalised and organised sport. Masculinity is fundamentally concerned with force, performance and competence, as is sport, such that displays of masculinity are designed to illustrate the 'natural' superiority of the male over females, or over other males (Connell 1983:28). Connell does not seem to mention, however, that sex itself, as in copulation or 'scoring', is a form of sport or competition among men. He does write, though, about the extent to which constructs of masculinity oppress women and become dysfunctional for men who do not define themselves within stereotypical masculine frameworks, or who do not possess the 'natural' physical prowess of maleness. Connell's (1983:27) analysis of masculinity is much less phallocentric in that he argues that 'genital potency is a specific organisation *within . . .*' a system where masculinity is embodied in force – the penis is an instrument through which that power is exercised.

Power, sexuality and masculinity

Belief in the 'natural' superiority of males over females, particularly in sexual matters, was a central idea in the work of Havelock Ellis (see Jackson 1984a), who became authoritative on these matters. He favoured an instinct-driven model of sexuality, resulting in a view which condoned existing constructs of male and female sexuality, and which provided grounds on which to argue that men had little conscious control over their sexual physiology. His view that courtship was a matter of conquering the female and her 'natural' modesty gave credence to the notion that the male was 'naturally' the aggressor in sexuality and that the female required (desired) pursuit (see Jackson 1984a, 1984b). He believed also that pain was normal and inevitable in sexual relations and that there was a 'normal' male instinct to use force (Jackson, 1984a:58). His ideas, in being phylogenetically reductive, provided a rationale for two enduring notions of male sexuality and sexual behaviour. Firstly, his model bestowed on human sexuality elements of animal behaviour more characteristic of lower species where learning does not have such influence on sexual behaviour as it does in humans. In so doing he absolved people of responsibility for the body in sexual relations. Secondly, his model separated mind and body, making it conceptually difficult to incorporate the social context of sexuality and sexual expression with biology.

While social scientists may have learned more about male sexuality, and the extent to which it is modified by learning and social processes, the ideas which Ellis promoted surface from time to time in media reports of rape (Walby et al 1983), in media generally (Dyer, 1985), and as a common theme in pornography (see for example Faust 1980, McNall 1983, Moye 1985, Eardley 1985). A telling illustration of these ideas is found in Hollway's (1987) account of media coverage of the trial of Peter Sutcliffe, the Yorkshire Ripper. She documented how reports from the trial and comments from trial lawyers and the judge attempted at times to portray him as a man driven by motives, including aggression, which were part of 'normal' male sexuality. However 'abnormal' they were, Sutcliffe's actions nevertheless presented a problem for the (mostly male) British press as it attempted to explain his difference from ordinary men. Hollway argues that the press, through the discourse of the trial, attempted to find a space in which to explain Sutcliffe's actions that did not render male sexuality itself problematic.

The patriarchal discourse sees as quite 'natural' a bit of aggression in men's sexuality . . . [and] to this extent Sutcliffe is normal. But what made him kill? Male sexual violence must be seen as a way of asserting 'masculinity' by exercising power over women. Sutcliffe's first murder came after a prostitute had accused him of being 'fucking useless' when he was slow to get an erection . . . . The ability to get an erection is the symbol of a man's masculinity, and it signifies his power (Hollway 1987:128–129).

The Sutcliffe case serves as an extreme example of motives and actions which are part of so-called 'normal' male sexuality, sexual behaviour and masculinity and it illustrates not only that power is integral to being male, but that such power is vested in the possession of a penis. Cameron and Frazer's (1987) analysis of the social bases of sexual murder (lust killings), including those committed by Peter Sutcliffe, illustrates the interrelated construction of masculinity and sexuality and how easily it slips into themes of power and violence in our culture. To them, 'sexuality does not stand apart from the rest of culture' but is a product of it, and in our culture male sexuality is typified by *'performance, penetration, conquest'* (Cameron & Frazer 1987:169) – all of which are penis-centred.

Another extreme illustration of the belief that masculine power resides in the penis is found in Tannahill's (1980:246–254) analysis of the roles and symbolic significance of eunuchs, who serve to demonstrate not only that the penis (and testes) is the symbol of power, but that the power to remove it (or the testes) is the ultimate form of dominance among males.

What is so interesting about the construction of male sexuality is that it stands in sharp contrast to rationality, which is also believed (by some) to be so characteristically masculine (see Keller 1983, Lange 1983, Lloyd 1984, Harding 1984). Rationality, which is itself believed to be innate in males in this view, is replaced in matters of a sexual nature by a plea that biology overtakes rationality. The defence of such male sexual behaviour then takes on the quality of 'I'm sorry, Your Honour, my penis made me do it'.

The primacy of the penis

In male sexuality and sexual behaviour, the penis is the primary focus of sexual experience whereas women's sexual orientation and experience is seen to be more diffuse, there is no one central physical feature which is the centre of sexuality. Dyer's (1985:29) analysis of media images of sexuality illustrate this because he found that

male sexuality is repeatedly equated with the penis; men's sexual
feelings are rendered as somehow being 'in' their penises. Sexual
arousal in women, where it is represented at all, may use a plethora of
indications — arching bodies, undulating shoulders, hands caressing
breasts, hips, arms, textures, and surfaces that suggest all this – such is
the vocabulary of female desire in the media.

According to Dyer (1985:30), male genitals are symbolised as weapons, frequently being represented by real weapons – 'swords, knives, fists, guns' while women's genitals are represented by such things as flowers. Rarely, he claims, are male genitals depicted as the fragile structures that they are, but as 'hard, tough, and dangerous' (Dyer 1985:30). His analysis also emphasises how the media depict the male as somehow the helpless victim of his penis, especially through such films as Percy in which the 'hero' is the captive of a grafted penis that assumes control of the host body. It is a form of biological determinism which is reserved for sexuality whereby the man is not responsible for what his body does – he has no control and, therefore, he is absolved of responsibility. This is an especially useful notion (for men) when one considers that the penis is the major symbol of male potency.

At best the man is seen as the possessor or owner of this object, but it is
an object over which he does not have full control. It is the beast below.
    The idea of the penis, and hence male sexuality, as separable from
the man, forms the basis of stories about male sexuality, especially those
with a violent or bestial view of sexual intercourse itself (Dyer 1985:31).

The primacy of the penis, and the felt need for it to become erect in order to establish masculinity, is illustrated in Tiefer's (1986) study of men seeking a surgical cure for impotence. Tiefer argues that to men who cannot get an erection the word 'impotence' is more than a simple description of a particular physiological event (or non-event). She claims that impotence is a highly stigmatising and stressful experience for some men because the ability to have an erection serves as a gender-confirming symbol. She compiled a list of what the literature indicated were 'the ten sexual beliefs to which many men subscribe' (1986:581) – all of which require erection. They are:

(1) Men's sexual apparatus and needs are simple and straightforward, unlike women's. (2) Most men are ready, willing, and eager for as much sex as they can get. (3) There is suspicion that other men's sexual experiences approximate ecstatic explosiveness more closely and more often than one's own. (4) It is the responsibility of the man to teach and lead his partner to experience pleasure and orgasm(s). (5) Sexual prowess is a serious, task-oriented business, no place for experimentation, unpredictability, or play. (6) Women prefer intercourse to other sexual activities, particularly "hard-driving" intercourse. (7) All really good and normal sex must end in intercourse. (8) Any physical contact other than a light touch is meant as an invitation to foreplay and intercourse. (9) It is the responsibility of the man to satisfy both his partner and himself. (10) Sexual prowess is never permanently earned; each time it must be reproven (Tiefer 1986:581).

Tiefer argues that, although impotence is frequently psychogenic, medical practitioners (who are mostly men) have not been slow to medicalise impotence by using surgical implants to alleviate what they see as a mechanical problem – the consequence of which is that the impotent man need no longer feel responsibility for what has become a 'medical problem'. Tiefer is extremely critical of this process, and claims, among other things, that the medicalisation of impotence leaves unquestioned the social meanings attached to male sexual performance. It also leaves unquestioned the phallo-centric nature of male sexuality and sexual expression and their relationship to the body.

There is an interdependence of masculinity, sexuality and the body which are bound together into a construct of sex/power/body. Person (1980:619) believes that, for men, masculine gender 'leans' on sexuality much more than is the case for femininity or female sexuality and that 'the relationship between genital sexuality and gender is . . . the single most telling distinction between female and male sexuality'. To be masculine is to empower the body sexually and simultaneously to use that power to express masculinity. Masculinity relies on a sexualised body, as Tiefer (1986) found in her study of impotent men.

There is widespread consensus that male sexuality is power oriented, that it is a construct in which the phallus (and its potential to become erect) is central if not essential, and that it is fundamentally corporeal in nature. It is different from female sexuality not only because it is power oriented and phallocentric, but also because it is conceptualised as less controllable and more proactive, if not aggressive. It is a construct which legitimises male control over women and male power among men. The man with the biggest penis among his colleagues has a status which his fellow men cannot share – he has proof of his superiority by virtue of one single biological structure. The penis is both a symbol and a source of power and it is the penis which demonstrates how biology and culture interact to contribute to the construction of masculinity and male power. Our language reflects these relationships as Greer (1971:41) and Hartsock (1984) demonstrate. The superiority that men assume over women is enacted through the body via its perceived power/masculinity/sexuality.

WOMEN'S BODIES AND EMBODIED EXPERIENCE

The female body is a problem for women in patriarchal society because it forms a nexus with reproduction and sexuality through which female roles are constructed and reinforced. Kupfermann (1979) began her book, *The MsTaken Body*, with this quote from Adrienne Rich: 'I know of no woman – virgin, mother, lesbian, married, celibate – whether she earns her keep as a housewife, a cocktail waitress, or as a scanner of brain waves – for whom her body is not a fundamental problem'.

Whereas the literature on men's bodies has emphasised the phallus, power and the nexus of the body, masculinity and sexuality, women's bodies have been articulated around different themes, such as inequality and oppression, sexual exploitation and lack of control over the body's reproductive ability. Feminists have written about how the female body, like the male body, is a central mechanism through which men exercise dominance over women in patriarchal systems. The body provides the medium through which women are exploited by men. In their writings on rape, pornography, abortion, birth control, the medicalisation of pregnancy, and other aspects of women's lives, feminists demonstrate that the female body and its sexualised nature are inscribed with social meanings which disadvantage women within patriarchy.

Where maleness has been discussed in terms of physical strength, power and genitalia, femaleness has been conceptualised within a gynaeco-dominant framework such that women are seen as victims of their own reproductive anatomy (see in particular Shorter 1984, Todd 1983, Tuana 1988a, 1988b). Female sexuality and the experience of being a woman are also fundamentally tied, in some minds, to physical qualities associated with women's reproductive organs and reproductive experience (Ferguson 1986). Women's bodies are conceptualised in terms which are consistent with female roles in society generally. For example, infertility is not only associated with biological (bodily) processes, it also interrelates with perceived 'natural' roles for women, including motherhood – a role which the press has promoted as 'normal' for women (Albury 1987).

Women's sexuality (that is, women's experiences of and others' perceptions of them as sexual beings), however, as opposed to the biological capacity for reproduction, has not been a subject of much enquiry, beyond the physiological, and the subject of female sexuality did not appear in the literature during the explosion of discourse on feminism in the 1970s (Rich 1986). Most attention has been on female experience and patriarchy, and it has been developed by studying rape, sexual assault, incest and domestic violence, and consequently the body and its relationship to power and patriarchy have remained relatively peripheral topics. However, because women's reproductive powers have been integral to their roles and to their oppression, particularly prior to the ready availability of birth control, feminists have long recognised the relationship between biology and culture when it concerns reproduction, maternity and motherhood. Again, however, the focus has tended to be on the structural aspects of a patriarchal society which victimises women because of their biology, and as a result the debate subsumes the body. The subject of women's bodies and the relationship to sexuality has not, therefore, been overtly studied or theorised until very recently.

Women's sexuality has become a popular subject of enquiry and discussion among feminists, although they have examined it indirectly for many years in relation to reproduction and birth control (see, for example, Cohen 1986, Petchesky 1986, Martin 1987, Caplan 1987, Lunbeck 1987, *Sexuality: A Reader* 1987 edited by *Feminist Review*, Hite 1988, Jaggar & Bordo 1989).

Sexuality is now being conceptualised as an aspect of embodied existence because it is simultaneously a biological and social activity involving the body. This is the sort of approach I have called somology, and which is illustrated in later chapters in discussions of the work of nurses. However, somology can also be used to understand sexuality by integrating understanding of the object body's physiological responses, existential experience of sexual encounters and the symbolic meanings associated with them. Because sexuality also involves social learning and practical knowledge it requires a framework which allows for personal knowledge.

Theorising women's bodies and female sexuality

Role theory, androgyny, and most recently, existentialism, have all been used as theoretical frameworks in which to locate analyses of women's bodies, female sexuality, and the experiences of embodied womanhood. Caddick (1986) gives an account of feminist sociologists' attempts to theorise women's bodies – attempts which she says suffer from an assumed dualism that disembodies women, resulting in precisely the opposite of what is intended. This is particularly the case in the work of those who adopted role theory. By emphasising role and self, the body is absent or silent; it has no place in explanations of gender difference based only on social constructs. Androgyny, however, which emphasises sameness and tends to make difference appear to be an artifact of the interface between biology and society, is also shown by Caddick to be inadequate. In this she is consistent with Elshtain (1981:11) who argues that '. . . the body is a prison for androgynists, [and] the female body is life imprisonment with torture to boot'.

Turner (1984:233), who also theorised the female body (and female sexuality as an aspect of embodied existence) in sociology, claims that women, like other oppressed groups such as slaves, have not enjoyed 'a phenomenological possession of their bodies' and rarely have they 'enjoyed full ownership', rather, their bodies have been commodified in legal and political systems which deny them ownership. Prostitution is but one example of this (see Perkins & Bennett 1985) as is the more recent trend toward technologised reproduction and invitro fertilisation in which women's reproductive capacity is commodified (Caddick 1987, Albury 1987).

Turner takes a predominantly structural and political stance for his analysis of women's bodies, although he recognises that interpretive and existential approaches are also necessary. It is the latter approach which is most common in recent feminist theorising, particularly among French feminists, such as Kristeva (1982) and Irigaray (1987). They approach the problem from a psychoanalytic/existential viewpoint which is not very helpful in an empirical approach and which does not easily integrate with non-psychoanalytic constructs of human nature and sexuality. To that extent this style of French feminist work on the body is limited, and limiting.

To Caddick (1986:68), the body represents a 'vacant space' in social theory. This view is shared by Rothfield (1986:157–158), who claims also that writing the (female) body into sociology will be 'a rather difficult prospect for feminism [because] ... this subject is ... also constituted by its lack'. Women have been studied in ways which make the problem of the body and sexuality central but never overt – in rape, pornography, fashion and abortion, for instance – all of which pivot on constructs of the female body.

Both Caddick (1986) and Rothfield (1986) reflect a growing trend in feminism to write the body into sociology, especially the subjective and existential body, but as they clearly see, this will be difficult because our current philosophical and epistemological constructs of consciousness, rationality and mind are heavily dualistic, and they reflect an organisation of knowledges which excludes some forms of knowing.

Germaine Greer (1971) was one of the earliest feminist writers, in *The Female Eunuch*, to articulate the female object body in patriarchy. It is work which is truly provocative because she makes the body so very explicit, particularly in her discussion of female sex organs. These organs are the most mysterious and deeply invested with symbolism, and they are more likely to be spoken of in pejorative terms than other parts of the female body.

The worst name anyone can be called is *cunt*. The best thing a cunt can be is small and unobtrusive: the anxiety about bigness of the penis is only equalled by anxiety about smallness of the cunt. No woman wants to find out she has a twat like a horse-collar: she hopes she is not sloppy and smelly, and obligingly obliterates all signs of her menstruation in the cause of public decency (Greer 1971:39).

Greer (1987a, 1987b) continued this 1971 theme with two essays on the ways in which women are encouraged to sanitise and deodorise their pudenda to make them more aesthetically pleasing.

It looks bad. Shave it. Pluck it. Cover it with your hand . . . . It smells bad. Wash it. Scour it. Douche it. DEODORISE it. It tastes bad. Wash it some more. It's sloppy. Mop it. It's dry. Lubricate it. . . .

> If you doubt that the cunt is hated and feared by most of the population how will you explain the hundreds of thousands of pounds spent in persuading women that they have an intimate deodorant problem?
>
> Up to twelve or thirteen pages are spent in every women's magazine in stressing that cunts smell bad, not just when dirty or menstruating, but all the time (Greer 1987a:74–75).

The female body and its relationship to sexuality, in Greer's (1971, 1987a) view, would appear to be more closely related to notions of pollution and contamination which Mary Douglas (1984) believes underlie the symbol system of any culture. But the meanings associated with being female and female sexuality in western culture seem to be associated with ambivalence and contradictions, all of which imply that there is something dangerous about the female body and female sexuality. And there seems no way of knowing how or why women's bodies and female sexuality should be constructed in this way and there has been little research in this area.

There have been some important recent attempts, though, to articulate the female body, especially through the experience of embodiment and its links to genderisation and sexualisation (Birke & Best 1980, Suleiman 1986, Haug 1987, Butler 1987, Grosz 1987, Matthews 1987, Kirby 1987, Celermajer 1987, Reiger 1987, Kroker & Kroker 1988a, Garvey 1987). It is a literature which grows daily and promises to be one avenue through which a sociology of the body can be explored, however, these works bring into focus the limitations of existing paradigms and the mystique of the body itself and its association with sexuality.

Beyond the aesthetic aspects of female genitalia there is the mystery which surrounds the uterus and menstruation. No other organ has been inscribed with such power as that of the uterus. Greer (1971) calls it 'the wicked womb' – a term which succinctly describes its place in western medicine, history, mythology, and women's lives. Throughout history, the particular workings of women's reproductive organs, and the uterus in particular, have been used, generally under the umbrella of 'science', to legitimise the exclusion of women from a wide range of social and political activities (Tuana 1988a, 1988b).

Women as victims of their bodies (uteruses)

The idea that women are victims of and 'naturally' weakened by their reproductive activities is not new. For example, Shorter's

(1984) book, *A History of Women's Bodies*, which is alleged to be an historical analysis of women and their bodies, amounts to little more than a history of the control the uterus had over women. His account chronicles women's birthing experiences in such a way that he too, though he denies it, is perpetuating the belief that women are victims of the uterus, and his book epitomises the gynaeco-dominant approach to women's bodies. That is not to say that childbirth was not, and is not, a potentially dangerous process, rather, it is a criticism of Shorter's approach, because it reduces women to the sum of their uteruses and reproductive capacities.

Menstruation, however, needs special mention and discussion because no body product has been so invested with symbolism as menstrual blood (Buckley & Gottlieb 1988). The place of menstruation in our language signifies its place – it is called 'the curse', or the more genteel 'periods', or the scientised 'menses' (Greer 1971:51–52), and its regular occurrence in the lives of women is secreted away from public view. Only in the last decade have the sanitary paraphernalia associated with menstruation been openly displayed on shop counters and sold in supermarkets and even more recently advertised on television. I remember as a budding feminist in the early 1970s attending a rally in Sydney's Hyde Park at which two women performed a small piece of street theatre involving several articles of the sanitary management of menstruation. They were arrested by two male police for indecent behaviour in a public place. Their arrest illustrated to all present that, at least in the view of the male police, some body functions should not be publicised.

Buckley and Gottlieb (1988:3) introduce the reader to their *Blood Magic: The Anthropology of Menstruation* by claiming that

for all the significance attributed to menstrual symbolism by anthropologists and others, and for all the fascination with which its origins and functions have been pursued, little has been firmly established. While menstruation itself has at least a degree of biological regularity, its symbolic voicings and valences are strikingly variable, both cross-culturally and within single cultures. It is perplexing, then, that the study of menstrual symbolism has been limited by a paucity of detail regarding such variations, by imbalances of ethnographic reporting, and by overly reductionistic theoretical frameworks.

These two authors further claim that what ethnographic work exists on menstrual customs has centred on the notion of taboos and pollution (Buckley and Gottlieb 1988:4) and that menstruation/menstrual blood is believed to be dangerous and/or offensive

(1988:6). They believe '"the menstrual taboo" as such does not exist' (1988:7) but that menstruation has multiple meanings, not all of them to do with danger and pollution. In short, customs associated with menstruation are as varied as cultures themselves.

There is evidence that within our western heritage menstruating women are a source of disgust, if not pollution, and that they must therefore be avoided (Showalter & Showalter 1970). For example, in the 1800s when the Contagious Disease Act provided for the compulsory examination of female prostitutes suspected of having venereal disease, some suspects were able to avoid inspection by claiming they were menstruating at the time. 'Disgusted and appalled, the magistrate usually dismissed the court immediately', but in 1869 the Act was amended and provided for five days detention of the suspect so that the allegedly menstruating woman could then be examined (Smith 1971:120–121). More recently it has been noted that menstruating women are never shown in pornographic films (Laws, cited in Bart et al 1985) which would seem to indicate that even the makers of pornography, where nothing seems taboo, ignore menstrual blood and the menstruating woman as subject matter.

In western culture, menstruation has been pathologised (Weeks 1981:42–43) and medicalised in keeping with our methods of explaining the world. Zita (1988:77) outlines a long list of studies which claim to establish pre-menstrual syndrome as a causal agent in such diverse behaviours as propensity to be violent and irritable, fantasise with morbid and sexual themes, commit suicide, take children to the doctor, break the law, take leave from work, batter children, over-indulge in alcohol, end marriages, crash aeroplanes, and so the list goes on. In a technological age we are replacing taboo and pollution symbols with those of medicine and pathology, but the process is not complete and it would be false to assume that our culture is without a degree of reserve about menstrual matters. We have multiple names for these things, we treat menstruation with relative secrecy, and we do not discuss such things in public, and certainly not in mixed company – at least not in 'civilised' society, but there are signs of change, as television advertising attests.

In summary, therefore, women's bodies are problematic to the extent that menstruation and other aspects of reproduction are mythologised, but Ruth (1987) argues that women are conceptualised as essentially carnal creatures, and that what makes them carnal centres on the mysterious and hidden nature of their sexual anatomy – menstruation and birth come from hidden places. If it is true, as Ruth suggests, that women are seen as essentially carnal creatures, then they will be conceptualised as essentially victims of their bodies, and this has a number of consequences. On the one hand, they can be seen as essentially sexual in nature, and much that one sees in popular culture would suggest that women are seen this way, at least in television advertising. Sexuality, as it is portrayed in media, takes on a particular bodily form in such taken-for-granted notions as a 'sexy body' or a 'cheeky bum'. Almost any part of the body or any behaviour can be sexualised so that it is possible to talk in terms of a 'sexy [any part of the body you care to mention]'. One can **be** sexy, **look** sexy, **act** sexy, **feel** sexy. But what ever form sexuality takes, it is essentially a corporeal entity. The body and sexuality are indivisible, the body is a sexualised construct which impacts on social life and vice versa, and it influences the ways people interact with each other. This is clearly illustrated in studies about which areas of other people's body it is socially permissible to touch.

BODY ACCESS, TOUCHABILITY AND TOUCH

In social relations certain things are taken for granted about what one does with one's body and how it is used (Mauss 1973), how it is dressed, which parts of it are exposed, and what one does to control its functions. There are also taken-for-granted rules about where, how, and when it is socially acceptable to touch other people. Some body parts are heavily proscribed, most are invested with some social meaning, and there are context-related considerations. Perkins and Bennett (1985:215) remark, for example, that 'if a prostitute touches genitals and "relieves bodily functions" ... she is considered perverted, sinful, dirty, but if a doctor touches genitals and relieves bodies this is therapeutic, a cure, a blessing', although the context is different and the nature of the touch (presumably) varies.

The role of the body in social relations has not been well researched and neither has it often been taken into account in anthropology (Douglas 1971). Douglas argues that

the body communicates information for and from the social system in which it is a part. It is itself the field in which a feedback interaction takes place. It is itself available to be given as the proper tender for some of the exchanges which constitute the social situation. And further it mediates the social structure by itself becoming its image (1971:387).

One way in which the symbolic meanings of the body and different body parts have been studied is the notion of 'body accessibility', which Jourard (1966:222) defined as a willingness to touch and be touched by others. Body access has also been examined indirectly in studies which have focused on how professionals who work on the body (medical practitioners in particular) manage the context of physical examination. There is also some work on the social aspects and experience of touch which is informative.

Body accessibility

A series of papers on body accessibility (Jourard 1966, 1967, Jourard & Rubin 1968) give some indication of the taken-for-granted meanings which are attached to various body parts and those which are inscribed with sexual meaning.

Jourard (1966) conducted some field observations in London, Paris, San Juan (Puerto Rico), one city in the United States and a university teaching hospital in Florida. He observed that there was little evidence of touch in Florida or London, in contrast to Paris and San Juan. He followed the field work with a questionnaire survey of 160 male and 140 female unmarried college students in Florida. They ranged in age from 18 to 22 years. He used two charts (adapted from the sort displayed in butchers' shops indicating different cuts of meat) showing the back and front of the human form, and asked his participants to indicate (anonymously) on the charts which areas of the body were seen (clad or unclad) and/or touched, and which parts of others they had seen (clad or unclad) and/or touched by each of four target groups — mother, father, closest friend of the opposite sex, and closest friend of the same sex. He reported that there was 'considerable laughter, and some embarrassment' over the nature of the task, but also a 'great deal of interest' (1966:223). Jourard found that: bodies are more visually accessible than they are in a tactile way, except for opposite sex friends; few parts of the body are touched if the target person is a parent or a friend of the same sex; relatively few parts are visualised; females are touched more than males; and there was a high degree of reciprocity in touch generally, in that those areas of the bodies of others which the subjects reported touching were also touched on their own bodies. Non-sexual regions of the body showed a very variable pattern of touchability generally, and the reported data show higher standard deviations in the scores for what is touched than for what is seen (mean standard deviations for touch and sight were 6.45 and 3.08 respectively).

There is clear evidence in Jourard's (1966) study that body parts associated with the biological functions of sexual intercourse have very low accessibility and touchability. Specifically, Jourard's results revealed that females never touch their father's genital area and only 2% of females reported touching the genital area of their mothers; females are much more likely to touch their father's breasts (reported 22%) than they are to touch their mothers' breasts (reported 6%). For males there was a similar pattern and only minor variations in percentage reports; they almost never touched their fathers' (reported 1%) or mothers' (reported 1%) genital areas and touched the breasts of their fathers (reported 23%) and their mothers (reported 8%) to much the same degree as for females.

Jourard hypothesises, among other things, that propensity to touch is possibly a feature of individual personality. However, there are patterns in his data which cannot be explained on a personality variable alone. For example, he observed that male children touched fewer regions on their parents' bodies than did female children, and that Jewish girls allowed fewer regions of their bodies to be touched than did Catholic or Protestant girls. Irrespective of the relationship, or the sex of the subject, the hands, followed by the forearms, were areas with high 'touchability'.

In the second and predominantly theoretical paper, Jourard (1967) reflected on his 1966 work and what it meant to young people of the 1960s. He argued that his research showed we are not a touch-oriented culture, rather, we are disembodied culturally, and that we touch very little, except in sexual contexts or contact sports. He suggests that this is an illustration of a repressive society where, as part of socialisation, we learn not to touch others and certainly not to touch others or ourselves in particular body regions.

Children who touch their own bodies, as in exploratory masturbation, are punished, and threatened with predictions of insanity and depravity. Children who touch other things (children encounter the world by means of touch) are slapped, and told 'mustn't touch'. They are taught to keep their bodies at a distance from things and people: look, but don't touch (Jourard 1967:661).

In a third paper Jourard and Rubin (1968) attempted unsuccessfully to demonstrate a relationship between self-disclosure and touching. It is a variation of Jourard's 1966 study and it shows the same pattern of body accessibility, or touchability. Again it shows that women are touched more than men are, that there is a high level of reciprocity in touch, and again there is virtually no reported touching of the genital area outside sexual encounters (and Jourard assumes here, as he did in his 1966 paper, that people are heterosexual).

Although Jourard's (1966, 1967) and Jourard and Rubin's (1968) work, which indicates what areas of the body it is 'safe' to touch, was done over 20 years ago, the data reported from my study will show that little seems to have changed. The genitalia, and especially the male genitalia, are the most difficult areas of the body for female nurses to touch. This is similar to the difficulties which Becker et al (1963:325) noted in their study of medical students who found that examining men's external genitalia was especially difficult in a social sense. However, patterns of who touches whom also relate to social status and gender.

Touch

According to Henley (1973), touch is another form of intimacy, which is interpreted differently by men and women; women do not interpret men's touch as sexual, but men interpret women's touch as sexual.

Montagu's (1978) work on touching, although it is heavily psychoanalytic, gives some indicators of the variable distribution of who touches which parts of another person's body. He argues that the English cultural tradition, which much of the western world inherited, is given to 'primness' and that this still remains to some extent. Montagu (1978:272) agrees with Henley that touch is another form of intimacy and 'a privilege usually granted only to those of one's own class or status whom one has allowed to pass across those social barriers which serve to exclude unprivileged'. It reduces social distance, it is often perceived as an invasion of one's privacy, and it can be interpreted as an exercise of power (Montagu 1978:273).

Nurses, therefore, must negotiate the cultural and status-bound aspects of social relations when they touch patients, and some of that touch necessarily involves handling parts of the body which are normally only touched in sexual contexts. Nurses must negotiate the taken-for-granted aspects of body accessibility, and at the same time violate those norms in doing what needs to be done with the body. In later chapters of this book interview data will be used to illustrate how nurses touch and handle other people's bodies in a way which is socially constructed as non-sexual and which minimises embarrassment. It requires personal and professional knowledge and skill that is learned by experience.

Touch in professional practice

Watson (1975) has theorised that there are two forms of touch: instrumental touch to assist in the performance of some act; and expressive touch which is a spontaneous and affective act. Nurses, she claims, use mostly instrumental touch, but that the 'genital regions of the body can be collectively thought of as a veritable "no man's land" (and no woman's land) so far as targets for touching are concerned' (Watson 1975:108). Generally, however, touch has not been popular as a subject for research in nursing and little is known about it (Weiss 1979) despite the considerable extent to which nurses touch others in performing nursing care. Some work is being done more recently in the area of therapeutic touch but it does not deal with the social management of touching that is under discussion here.

In a theoretical paper on touch Barnett (1972) argues that touch is a risky act in nursing, because of possible misinterpretation, and because being touched can increase anxiety in some people. McCorkle (1974) found that seriously ill patients were touched less than those in a fair to good condition, but she gives little information on how or where the patients were touched.

For nurses and other health workers, touching patients requires a particular manner and context to ensure that the act of touch is not misinterpreted. The context in which medical practitioners physically examine and touch patients has been studied by several researchers. Parsons (1951:451–452) claims that all forms of body contact are highly regulated, including exposure of the body and body contact, such that things like vaginal and rectal examinations would not normally be allowed outside a medical context. The act of undressing for a medical examination is also highly regulated and context-related. The medical practitioner does not normally remain in the room and watch a patient undress, but leaves or ensures privacy in some way and resumes the consultation with the patient disrobed and waiting for examination. In this any suggestion of sexually defining the situation is deliberately excluded, rather, the encounter is constructed as a professional event.

Emerson's (1971) work on sustaining the contextual definition of the situation during vaginal examination is a particularly graphic analysis of the importance for all parties of continuing to define the situation in the same way. The data which follow in this book confirm the same elements of successful social management of an otherwise highly unusual and embarrassing event that Emerson identifies: the need for all parties to define the situation as a professional encounter; the 'matter-of-fact' manner of the staff; the careful use of language; the need for context-related props that help construct the situation; avoidance of overly exposing the part to be examined; the air of detachment; the use of humour to minimise potential embarrassment; and the clear expectation that the patient and staff will behave 'properly'. Each of these elements and others which emerged in this study, will be discussed in detail in later chapters.

THE BODY, SEXUALITY, ACCESS AND TOUCH: A SUMMARY

The body and sexuality are intimately interrelated but there are important differences between the sexes which are reflective of patriarchy and a culture which is not comfortable with issues relating to sexuality and the body. This lack of comfort is demonstrated in language, our perceived 'need' to control the body and sexuality, in our inability to adequately incorporate sexuality and the sexualised body in theoretical knowledge, and in how we do or do not allow the body to be touched by others.

While it is possible for the body to be comprehensively sexualised, the difficulty in social life seems to lie in how the meaning of sexuality is shared between men and women. If male and female sexuality are not different facets of a continuum, and if male sexuality is a different construct from female sexuality, and if the two are not complementary, then there is room for considerable social conflict about what sexuality actually means, and what it means to behave in a sexually appropriate way. The literature suggests that male sexuality is problematic for women, and probably also for some men, to the extent that it embodies power, and power is essentially about the control of others. Female sexuality, as a relatively passive notion, would appear to be complementary to male sexuality, but only if one takes a functionalist view. And even if one takes a functionalist view, which would seem to be conceptually neat, it does not take account of the sexual exploitation of women. The evidence would suggest to me that male and female sexuality, constructed as they are around notions of embodied maleness and femaleness, reflect a wider social system which is patriarchal and oppressive to women.

Despite the differences between the sexualised male body and the sexualised female body, there is some evidence that the bodies of both males and females are invested with taken-for-granted rules about which parts it is socially permissible to touch and see, and in this there is consistency – the genital area is taboo to touch unless the context is sexual. This construction of the sexualised body, therefore, is problematic for an occupation such as nursing where sustained and invasive, but non-sexual touch, is integral and fundamental to nursing care. Part II of this book is a discussion of how some nurses manage those problems, the nature of nurses' work with respect to body care, how it has been theorised and taught, and the need to violate social boundaries and touch the bodies of others, including those body regions which are not normally accessible in public. As part of their work, nurses must negotiate not only normal social boundaries when they touch others (patients), but, because the body is heavily inscribed with meaning – much of it sexual – nurses' work is socially fragile, and they must learn ways to make their work manageable.

Somological Practice

Sociological Practice

5. Body care and learning to do for others

This chapter, which is the first of a series which draws on the empirical data from the interviews and field work, describes how the participants' personal backgrounds influenced their first and early experiences of performing body care for patients, what they found difficult in carrying out that care, and the impact of the reality of nursing and its occupational subculture on their early experiences. This chapter and Chapter 6 provide the broad general background against which to view the body and body care in nursing practice.

Nursing care requires access to every part of the body which is potentially touchable. However, as Chapter 4 outlined, in western cultural traditions, certain parts of the body are more (socially) accessible and more readily touched than other parts. We are culturally 'non-touching' and this is especially so for the British. As nurses learn how to perform their work, therefore, they must overcome their own socio-cultural backgrounds and adjust to a particular professional subculture and its established methods that permits handling other people's bodies. They must also confront the symbolism of certain parts of the body, in particular, parts which have sexual significance, and they must find ways to manage social interaction during those times when they break taken-for-granted rules about the body.

The people whose experiences are discussed in this study come mostly from families with British backgrounds or families with some British influence, predominantly English, Irish, and some Scottish (in that order). Although most people in the sample described themselves as 'Australian', they were able to identify ethnic influences on family attitudes and practices associated with nakedness, body exposure, and acceptable topics of conversation about the body. It was reasonable to assume, therefore, that they would have found some of their first experiences of working with other people's bodies to be socially awkward. Coming as they did from a non-touching cultural background, many of the nurses I talked with found that they were, among other things, acutely embarrassed in having to perform body care for others.

It is generally the case that those who had the least difficulty touching and handling the bodies of patients came from backgrounds with a relatively relaxed attitude to the body and exposure (but they were few in number) or had friends or family who were nurses (and there were few of them). Most of the interviewees described a style of family life and upbringing where body functions were dealt with in a 'civilised' manner (see Elias 1978). The sensitive bodily functions were carried out in private and they were not discussed. The body was almost always kept covered, consistent with the established cultural patterns of their families, and this socialisation was acknowledged as a difficulty for a beginning nurse, as one nurse explained.

I.   *I can remember the first man I had to wash. That was traumatic . . . . I was timid. I was embarrassed, I guess. The women weren't quite so bad, I mean that was a shock but a different sort of shock to the men.*
R.   *Why are the men worse?*
I.   *I had never seen men naked and – even though I had brothers – three brothers. I mean you were just very modest, I guess, when you were at home.*
R.   *So you came from a family who kept things covered up?*
I.   *Oh yes.*
R.   *Did they talk about bodily functions?*
I.   *No, see they were very English in that respect. They were something that you didn't talk about. Nothing like that was.*
R.   *So when people went to the loo?*
I.   *It was behind a closed door and that was it.*
R.   *Did that make it very difficult for you as a nurse to then have to do for others what was [taboo], in your family life?*
I.   *Taboo. Yes, I guess so, yes.*

Among those I interviewed there was considerable individual difference in their reactions to first performing nursing care which involves touching the body, and this is due not only to their family upbringing, but also to how they were initially introduced to nursing practice. There are other factors, however, that influence these experiences, and they have their origins in the way the body is constructed in our culture. In particular the relationship of maleness and male power to genitalia and sexuality had a powerful effect on some of the female interviewees. The power invested in the male body is a theme which recurs throughout this study. The first experience of doing body care for others was often also the first introduction to what nurses' work really involved, and many of those I interviewed felt unprepared to deal with it because it was unfamiliar.

FIRST EXPERIENCE OF BODY CARE FOR OTHERS

While much has been written to educate nurses, nurses' own experiences of learning about body care, like nurses' experiences generally, are not well researched. Nurses are also poorly prepared, educationally, for the breaking of social norms which many nursing acts necessarily involve. What they learn of these things they learn through experience.

We are taught the proper way to carry out a bed bath, but not how to deal with the breaking of the social taboos when we wash a patient's body. Most nurses remember the fear they felt when doing their first bed bath. As a young female you work with a patient (who might well be male), behind drawn curtains and are expected to strip and wash his whole body. I remember feeling shamed and confused; my hands felt stiff, cold, awkward and useless. A bed bath can be embarrassing for the patient at the best of times – but far worse when the nurse herself [sic] is embarrassed (Berry 1986:56).

Berry's experience is mirrored by that of the people interviewed for this study. They talked of feeling terror, embarrassment and timidity when they first had to confront other people's nakedness, and at having to undress people, particularly men.

Normal male-female relationships in society are disrupted in nursing, especially when a beginning female nurse encounters her first male patient. She has not yet learned the interpersonal skills that will later make her work manageable. While male nurses experience some feelings of embarrassment when they encounter female patients for the first time, the data reported here suggest their discomfort is not as acute. It is possible, however, that my data reflect what men were willing to tell a woman about their sense of discomfort and also what women are prepared to discuss with another woman (see Warren 1988).

For many, sponging a patient for the first time was highly significant, and they have retained vivid memories of that occasion. They acknowledge it as a major milestone – a time when the reality of nursing confronts them. After the first sponge, however, doing body care for others seems to become much easier. In recent decades nurses have learned basic skills, such as how to sponge patients, during a period of initial instruction called, among other things, PTS (preliminary training school). Some nurses in this study, however, did not have such a period of instruction under supervision.

I asked each of the interviewees if they could remember the first time they had to 'do for someone else what that person would normally do for themselves'. Almost without exception they related stories of the first time they had to sponge a patient. Because it was a relatively common practice for nurse educators to introduce beginning students to body care with the subject of sponging, it would be expected that some remember the event for this reason. There are, however, other aspects of their memories which stem from our culture's approach to the body, male-female relations in our society, and to the reality of nursing – a reality which includes undressing and washing men's bodies.

The naked male body

In many of the accounts I heard from female nurses there was an early sense of profound embarrassment, lack of social competence and sometimes fear associated with men and having to deal with male bodies, particularly when the genitalia are exposed. It is an aspect of nursing practice which is often surrounded by social awkwardness and uncertainty. The following accounts indicate the early discomfort and fear of having to deal with the naked male:

*Yes. I can [remember my first experience with body care]. We went in PTS to Ward 5, . . . this **long** pavilion ward – a **men's** ward. [I] begged not to go to a men's ward first. Anyway, [I] went to the men's ward . . . . Went to the men's ward. Didn't want to go there. Would have done anything but go to the men's ward for sponging. Didn't want to go there. Anyway, went there, and was terrified through the whole procedure . . . . Just was terrified . . . . I remember it really clearly. . . . Women did not worry me. Men worried me a lot.*

******

I copped Male Ward. And I had to go to the corner [bed] – a boy about 18 he was. And he had a plaster on his leg, and so I gave him the dish and told him to wash himself, and he wasn't going to take his underpants off, and I wasn't about to take them off either! (Laughter) I can remember that as plain as day! . . . Oh, I was embarrassed. I don't know if I'd have handled it better if it was an old man. I certainly would have handled it better if it had been a woman. I was reared with three brothers too. Well, I just couldn't – I washed his back, and I washed his leg. But, there was no way I was going to tell him to take his underpants off! (Laughter) And I think that he was embarrassed and so was I. . . . I had seen men before, but to me, it wasn't –

*we'd been reared, you know, you don't look at men. And that to me was just
a problem. I was too embarrassed. . . . I still remember it as clear as day.*

★★★★★★

I can remember the very first day on the ward . . . **begging** *that they let me
do a female one [sponge] first because I couldn't bear the thought of pulling
down a pair of man's trousers. At that stage I don't think it even occurred
to me that my father had genitals. I was that protected from the male
anatomy . . .*

The first sponge is often the very first clinical act which beginning
nurses perform where the body is completely exposed, and where
they touch socially proscribed parts of the body. As the accounts
illustrate, the male genitalia are especially problematic and many
were very reluctant to touch those areas, as one would expect in a
society where the male sex organs are invested with such meaning
and kept covered, and where body contact in the genital areas is
almost exclusively reserved for sexual contexts. In the absence of
learned skills to manage these situations, the beginning nurse feels
socially awkward and embarrassed.

Some interviewees remember their first experiences as occasions
where they first saw suffering, disfigurement and death. And like
the naked body, one does not normally encounter these things
extensively in one's daily life, nor are they necessarily discussed in
detail, and even within hospitals there is a limit to what the public
sees, or is allowed to see or know. For some beginning nurses,
therefore, the first experience of body care was a first encounter
with male genitalia and nursing reality more generally — an
encounter which is sometimes shocking because of how little they
had known of nursing work.

Nursing reality

The work of nurses is not easily made public because it is invisible,
designated 'dirty work', and concerns privatised bodily functions.
As a consequence, neophyte nurses cannot know in detail what to
expect on their first encounters with the real world of nursing
practice. For some of those I interviewed, the first experience of
'doing for' is remembered because they came face-to-face with that
nursing reality.

*Yes. It [my first experience] sticks in my mind. I was sponging a person for
the first time. . . . It was a little old lady who'd had a stroke and was all bent
up . . . – so deformed.*

★★★★★★

It was a bit – I was a bit, um, hesitant (laughter) at first. [It was] the first time I saw someone laying in bed – they were just like a skeleton, you know. And we had to sponge them. Barely touch them and things like that. A bit scarey. . . . She looked so frail, didn't know how I could handle her. Didn't want to hurt her or anything. It wasn't the fact that she was naked or anything. That didn't bother me. I could handle that.

******

I can remember having to clean old men up for the first time. I'd never seen a man naked or anything like that before. You can imagine at [X Hospital] you had a lot of deros [derelicts] and that, and probably – I remember one guy being really filthy and smelt – the smell was unbelievable ... and that was horrible.

These accounts highlight the socially awkward nature of doing, for the first time, something as personal and private as washing the body of another person – a person who is a stranger to the nurse. The interviewees were also often shocked by what they were expected to manage as beginning nurses. Although they may have been instructed in doing various body care procedures, it was not usual for them to have any preparation or instruction in how to manage socially what those procedures entailed, nor how they might respond emotionally to what they had to do. The way(s) in which nurses have been (formally) instructed to carry out various body care procedures, and the particular work context in which nurses function, impact on individual experience, and that is illustrated in the accounts of the nurses who were interviewed. There is little need to comment on such accounts, because the interviewees' descriptions are graphic enough.

I remember it as vivid as anything. It was my first day in this big ward – ward 3. It was a great big medical ward like you'd have – about 36 patients. ... A Nightingale ward. Anyhow we were all going to the wards just for an evening, I think it was three hours or so, and I went to do something for this lady and I realised – she must have been – I thought she was dead – I couldn't get her to move, and I had to help the senior nurse lay her out, and that's the first time I had ever seen a dead body in my life. And that was an experience for me. . . . Never seen a dead body before in my life. I had to help this senior nurse sponge her, and I can remember sort of waking up with this face looking at me for a few weeks. I would say that was traumatic.

******

In the very early stages in PTS . . . they took us over to the hospital – it was one of those old Nightingale wards . . . . It was a male medical ward and there was a guy in a bed near the office and he was obviously on his last legs. Now I had had nothing to do with death except seeing my grandmother who was . . . very unwell but she wasn't unconscious, she was a bit delerious. This guy in the bed was, you know, vomiting blood, and the whole ward was like

*a zoo, and I walked in with one of my mates in PTS and I thought 'my
God, what have I got myself in for?' . . . and we had this guy who was in a
single room, you know, he was Cheyne-Stoking and he died. When he died
we looked at each other and said 'God, what are we gonna do now? He's
dead'. . . . We thought he was dead. We weren't real sure. We weren't real
sure. We kept saying to each other 'is he [dead]? Is he?' Well, we were sort of
hysterical with laughter for a while because we thought 'yeah, well he is dead
'cause that dreadful noise had stopped', but then we got sort of sad because we
hadn't witnessed anything like this before . . . .*

Other nurses remembered their first experiences because, as
beginners, they were disorganised, they lacked skill and they
encountered scenes for which they were completely unprepared.
As a consequence they felt inadequate. It is important for nursing
students to feel a sense of competence in their actions (Davis 1968)
and without it they feel unable to adequately convey a sense of
being in control – a sense that is needed in order to promote a
particular context in which to perform highly intimate care for
patients. The following two accounts, given by nurses who are now
very experienced and skilled at their practice, illustrate their felt
lack of competence – a lack which meant they had not yet developed
the occupationally specific methods that they could later use to
manage such situations. Speed is often used by nurses as a method
by which difficult things are managed, particularly those things
which are potentially embarrassing. The first account was given by
a male registered nurse, now in his 30s and skilled at care for
acutely ill and intensive care patients.

*I can remember we went to the ward, and . . . I can remember lining up with
all the bits and pieces, the bowl and stuff and thinking to myself 'I haven't
got a bloody clue what I'm doing here'. We'd done it on models and dummies
and that in the school but never actually done it on a person and I looked at
the man I was about to sponge. I can remember him, he was a big man, fat
man, and he'd had a cholecystectomy. He had an I.G. tube and he had a
drain in and a drip and I thought 'where will I start with all this – how will
I get the pyjamas off?' – that sort of stuff. I was slow. I know it took me 55
minutes . . . and even then I forgot to do things like clean his teeth and do all
that sort of thing. I was so intent on getting him washed. It was awful. . . . I
knew to wash him, and I knew what I had to do as far as washing and
drying and all that sort of thing, but not having any idea of the organisation
– and being slow. And it was hard because he knew that we were new.*

★★★★★★

*I have often had that woman's situation in my mind since. You know, it's
something I have not lost through the years, was going into a bathroom and
seeing this elderly lady in a bath and seeing her arm and leg floating on top
and she was weeping and couldn't express anything, and I later discovered
she'd had a stroke and she was aphasic. She had been a doctor, and you*

know how stroke people cry, and she just cried and cried, and couldn't express herself and it was sort of a trauma to me that I have never really lost. I can remember her, and I think that's a terrible thing – for a woman like that to come to that state and – I mean she couldn't move anything, her leg and arm were floating on top and the nurses were trying to bath her in a bath, and she was just crying and drooling and couldn't speak. . . . It was 'whatever do I do, whatever do I say?'

LEARNING 'BASIC' NURSING

When these nurses were taught how to do body care for others, it was in a particular manner – a manner which incorporated an emphasis on routine and procedure which involved no unnecessary exposure of the patient's body and which followed the recipe book approach characteristic of the texts. Additionally, the patient's embarrassment was to be considered, and nurses were also taught to maintain 'privacy' – a term which has a particular meaning where body care in nursing is concerned. Privacy has to do not only with avoiding unnecessary exposure, but it is also a notion about the vulnerability of patients. Instructions on clinical procedures emphasise privacy as a central consideration, along with the adherence to routine. This ritualised procedure, however, was constructed with an implicit somological approach to the extent that the nurse was to pay much attention to social management of the body by protecting the patient's 'privacy' and by guarding against potential embarrassment. The protection for the patient, however, seems to inhere in how the nurse goes about the procedure.

The emphasis on procedure

The accounts I heard in this study confirmed that nursing procedures, as they are described in texts, as step-wise and relatively stereotyped affairs, are indeed what nurses are taught as students. I asked those I interviewed how they had been taught to perform body care, especially sponging, which is the most central and comprehensive act of body care.

I.   *They [the teachers] were very strict, very 'thorough' – the word is.*
R.   *But what did they teach you about how you might socially manage things like other people's nakedness, and embarrassment, and modesty?*
I.   *I don't think they ever prepared you for that.*
R.   *So they taught you how to do the procedure . . . .*
I.   *Physically do it, yeah. By the book! It was a procedure.*

******

Yes, I can remember exactly what they [the nurse teachers] told us. Things they were more worried about were putting the sheets and the blankets in the right place and the towel in the right place and they never mentioned anything about how you should cope with the person, or the person coped with you. That was never, ever mentioned.

Others remembered being taught about a procedure which incorporated the notion of privacy, and how one might achieve this during the procedure. Privacy in this sense means not over-exposing the patient, and it also means ensuring a visual privacy such that others cannot see the patient's nakedness. In effect, it is dealing with the body in a privatised and 'civilised' way, but it is also somological – the nurse must 'do for' the body while simultaneously recognising personhood. The procedure, though, was dominant in their early formal education.

We were always taught to screen the patient and we were always taught about privacy – privacy as in 'from the rest of the ward' – to screen the patient and make sure we were in this little closed off area. We were taught nothing about embarrassment as far as the patient was concerned with the nurse. We were always taught to keep the patient warm which presumably meant you kept them covered, but then in the middle of summer you didn't need to be covered to be warm. We were always taught to keep them covered and taught to sponge by moving the sheet up and down various parts of the body – that sort of thing. . . . Exposing one bit at a time, but then at the same time we had to expose other bits, but nothing was ever talked about as far as patients' embarrassment or nurses' embarrassment. We were taught about privacy but it was privacy as in screening the patient from everyone else in the ward. . . . There was nothing about privacy between the nurse and the patient. It was always just there . . . .

******

R. *Can you remember ever getting any sort of instruction as a student nurse in how you might deal with someone else's naked body or body products.*
I. *Yes, you covered it up.*
R. *What was the function of covering it up?*
I. *Maintaining their privacy, that was one thing that I remember – all through PTS, all through training – 'maintain the patient's privacy!'*
R. *Were you given any instruction in how you might behave during this?*
I. *No.*

It would be false, however, to assume that this style of instruction is indicative of the way(s) in which nursing is practised in clinical settings. I have recorded elsewhere (Lawler 1984) that nurse educators often promote and teach nursing procedures in idealised and unrealistic ways that do not reflect clinical reality, or knowledge derived from clinical experience. Any detailed discussion of the reasons for this are beyond the scope of this study, however, it is important to establish that the knowledge nurses accumulate in practice does not readily lend itself to classroom style teaching with beginners, and it is not easily reduced to a level where neophytes can grasp it. What is important about these notions from the point of view of this study is that the ways in which nurses deal with the body in practice is implicit in the discipline, and, like other aspects of nurses' work and women's work, they have not been made overt and explicit either in research, education or discourse.

LEARNING TO CONTROL EMOTIONS

Much of what nurses' (women's) work entails, represents what Hochschild (1983) has termed 'emotional labour' – a commodification of feelings to suit the public (paid) arena. And emotions have largely been ignored by social science. Nurses are heavily involved in emotional labour because, as well as learning physically and procedurally how to wash another person in bed, there is an expectation that students will learn to control their emotions. Such emotional control is part of the nurse's 'professional' approach, that is learning how to do body care and perform other nursing functions in a manner typical of the occupation.

Many aspects of nursing have changed since it embraced the concept of individualised patient care described in Chapter 1. One such change is the recognition that some emotions are normal, if not desirable, and that it is probably not healthy for nurses (or anyone else for that matter) to suppress some emotions. Historically, however, one characteristic of a 'good' nurse, was the ability to hide emotional reactions and to cultivate an air of detachment – a sort of professional distance from one's work. Many of the nurses I interviewed remember being expected to learn such emotional control and to learn it as they developed their nursing skills, and as they coped with a daily working life that was often difficult and disturbing.

One British nurse, who is now in her 50s, described what she had been taught as a student nurse.

I don't think we had very much at all on relating to people as individuals. . . . You have to remember I'm British and the British stiff upper lip. . . . I think it was just that it was not done. It was not done for the nurse to show emotion . . ., it was to do with being professional and it upset the relatives. . . . I think it had to do with being a professional person. . . . [and] we learnt it because I think if you showed any emotion you couldn't cope as a nurse – you weren't made of the right stuff (laughter). You weren't suitable if you showed emotion. . . . We certainly didn't look sad, I mean, you were not allowed to look sad or grieve, but neither were you allowed to giggle around the place. You had to comport yourself – with dignity. . . . No frivolity, not at all.

With experience and more generalised social change, many nurses re-evaluate those early influences, particularly as they affect the ways in which they help patients come to terms with illness experience and the lived body. The ability to control emotion is often used by experienced and expert nurses as one method to help patients through illness experience, and that will be discussed in more detail in the following chapter. It is also useful, however, to examine how the secondary socialisation of nursing and the ethos of 'professionalism' as it was promoted in past decades affected nurses when they were attempting to overcome their primary socialisation as members of a 'civilised' society.

Other nurses, who are much younger than the British nurse whose experience is related above and who trained in Australia, relate similar experiences to those of their British colleague. The occupational ethos of emotional control remains relatively pervasive.

You were never allowed to [show emotion] – and you were never allowed to cry. You were only allowed to cry if the Charge Sister let you cry. (Laughter) You weren't allowed to cry if someone died or was really sick, you just felt that you had to give a little bit more to the patient – and you weren't allowed to laugh either if you could see the funny side of things . . . . You had to appear what they termed 'professional' which was very cold and caught up.

★★★★★★

We weren't taught about . . . emotions . . . and you weren't taught . . . that it's normal to feel disgust or things like that, which it is, isn't it. You know, you have a job to do and you do it, but no, not enough emotion or feeling was put into it.

★★★★★★

[I was] always told not to get involved and become attached to the patient or – it's hard not to get involved, I mean you do get involved. . . . I think it gets passed down, you know when you're looking after a really sick patient [other nurses say to you] 'you shouldn't get involved, you know' and so it goes on.

★★★★★★

I.   *No! No! No! It was never ever taught . . . that you would feel unhappy or uncomfortable about a situation. It was never taught.*
R.   *It was never what you could call a legitimate topic of conversation?*
I.   *No. Never. Never. It was like tears.*
R.   *Yes, you weren't allowed to have them.*

I.   No, there were many things that were taboo and that did not, therefore, require talking about. So . . . permission, so to speak, was never given to feel or [have] any emotional charge one way or the other. . . . . Feelings weren't allowed, there was no place for them really, so probably some feelings don't really emerge unless they are allowed to, you just find other ways of dealing with it.

Emotional control, as an ideal aspect of professional practice is now being seriously evaluated in the research literature. Benner & Wrubel (1988), for example, claim that it is impossible for nurses to care about what happens to patients and to help them during illness experience unless some degree of involvement occurs. Many of the nurses in my study would agree because they have recognised that emotional detachment does not work and that in some cases they have had to un-learn what had previously been taught to them.

I don't know whether they [your teachers] expected it [emotional control] to help you through your training or your working years, but it definitely didn't. And I find now that I'm trying to get back to the stage where – it's a hard process – you do think of them [patients] as people, and you don't classify them.

******

I think probably we were taught that [emotional control] to start, but I think I've learnt over the years that that isn't always appropriate to the occasion, that there are times when I think . . . that as a person I have the right to let that other person know that they are embarrassing me . . . or that I feel uncomfortable in a situation. . . . I think that's improved. I think once upon a time you weren't expected to be emotional about anything. We weren't expected to feel emotion if a patient we cared about or cared for died . . . . Now I think it's quite acceptable for the staff to be just as emotional about the situation as the family is. I think that's good. I think it's important that we let the people we're caring about know – that we really do care, . . . – you can't do that if you remain detached. Looking back I think that in our early training – that we were sort of expected to be a bit remote, you know [we were told] 'don't be silly, Nurse. Pull yourself together'.

******

Oh God yes [I was taught to be detached]! Never sit on the bed! Don't do this! Don't talk to them [patients]! That's a lot of bullshit. . . . .

The structured style that characterises instruction in body care procedures, and the occupational ethic of emotional control seem, on one level, to be a reflection of the British cultural traditions that are heavily embedded in much nursing ideology, and more widely in the culture. It is possible, for example, to trace direct links from contemporary nursing procedures to the early days of modern nursing in Britain in the mid-1800s. The procedural and ritualistic nature of such practices assists in the management of nurses' work because it allows the casting aside of normal social conventions about seeing people naked, undressing people and touching the bodies of others. It also provides the nurse with a focus for concentration that excludes the social rules which are being broken.

Wolf (1986b) argues that some nursing acts are conducted as rituals in order to make events socially manageable. Wolf's account, however, fails to consider the extent to which nurses choose not to follow standard procedures, nor how experience teaches them to ignore occupational practices which are impractical or dysfunctional in certain situations.

The notion of ritual, as the sole explanation for how nurses manage the body, is inadequate because it implies, at least in Wolf's terms, a form of social determinism which is not reflected in the accounts of nurses in this sample. Many of these accounts illustrate the extent to which, with experience, nurses modify what they have been taught and how they devise strategies specifically to deal with situations their instructors ignored. For example, they were not taught how to respond affectively in clinical practice other than to suppress what ever they felt, but lack of affect can be a very useful clinical tool.

Lack of affect as a clinical strategy

Nurses were expected to be controlled – to show no emotion. Many of them interpreted this to mean that they were to be emotionless, but lack of affect is in itself a response – a way of dealing with what would otherwise be a social mistake, a deviant act, an affront, an insult, a source of embarrassment. To show no affective change, for example, at another person's naked body, is a way of conferring a very different meaning on nakedness from the usual effect of running naked across the field at a sports event. While lack of affect is an everyday response of nurses, it is never made explicit as a way of dealing with the body but it is a very useful and successful strategy that is fundamental to dealing with clinical problems somologically.

Lack of affect is a means by which nurses construct context, so in that sense it serves to assist in the management of otherwise potentially embarrassing situations. The problem for nurses, however, is that lack of affect can become **the** standardised and expected emotional response, in which case it excludes the possibility of sharing difficult moments for patients in a way which allows the nurse to 'make contact' with the patient existentially (see Benner & Wrubel 1988:Ch.1).

In many ways nurses operate in a social vacuum because, as neophytes, they are often naive or ill-informed (at best) about the work they are expected to do and how they can behave, and little, if anything, in their lives prepares them for what they are required to do for others as basic nursing (body) care. Much of what nurses do is not public to protect patients' 'privacy', and it takes time and experience to feel comfortable in the role of nurse, doing things for other people. Talking with patients about some things is also difficult because there is a problem with language. Not only is it not always socially appropriate, or acceptable, to discuss what nurses do (as will be described in Chapter 10), there is a real difficulty choosing appropriate words or simply having conversation about various things to do with the body. This part of the data presented here, is richly indicative of 'the problem of the body' and privatised body functions and it highlights the silence of the body in discourse generally.

THE PROBLEM OF LANGUAGE

I asked the interviewees what they found most difficult to do when they first began nursing, and while many found the physical and procedural aspects of caring for other people's bodies awkward, there was a very real problem with language and conversation. Nurses were taught to explain always what they were going to do to patients, because patients are often unaware of what could happen during a certain procedure. For one nurse, this first experience of explanation is remembered very clearly.

In PTS . . . we were taken into the hospital one evening and assigned patients that we were to . . . sponge, and I was given an elderly gentleman who was virtually semi-conscious. I wasn't frightened so much of washing him, I was frightened of the fact that here was this man who was virtually non-responsive and I . . . remember going through all the motions we had been taught in PTS (laughter) — 'Mr. Bloggs, I'm just going to wash your hands and face', and Mr. Bloggs (laughter) didn't even care. . . . I don't remember ever feeling any embarrassment about washing him at all. The only embarrassment I can remember feeling was about talking to this person (laughter) who didn't respond. (Laughter) . . . This moribund man . . . probably went to God with my words ringing in his ears (laughter) – 'I'm just going to wash your feet now'. But I was so naive and terrified and frightened that . . . all I can remember was that, not that he was a man and I had to wash him, but I parroted my way through what I'd been taught in PTS. Looking back afterwards it was ridiculous and I felt a fool.

The need to explain indicates a number of things. Firstly, it is a basic method which nurses use in order to structure encounters with patients and which therefore assists in creating a context of, and defining the situations as, nursing care (of which more will be described in the following chapter). Secondly, it shows that some aspects of nursing care are not widely understood. Thirdly, nursing care is an interactive social affair which requires management to gain co-operation from the patient. In many of the accounts which follow, the notion of explanation recurs frequently and in relation to many aspects of nurses' work. The need to explain so frequently, and about so many things, is further evidence that much nursing work is invisible to the public. Explanation, however, is not straightforward because: firstly, some people are not relaxed about discussing some body functions or body parts; and secondly, the choice of words is far from straightforward. The two accounts below illustrate some of the general aspects of this problem. I had asked the interviewees if they found it difficult to know what to say to people when they were doing nursing care.

Embarrassing. Didn't know what to look at, what to say, because at those times I was quite shy and I can remember it was an old lady . . . with a fracture and . . . we had to . . . sponge and we had to do the whole works not knowing what to say or what to touch when you got to those bits . . . because it's something you don't ask . . . . We didn't know if that person would be offended by what we said. If you said 'your boobs' would she be offended by that. Being older she would probably be a bit strict.

******

*We were never taught how to deal with that [the language difficulty]. I mean, to ask a patient if they wanted to wash, for example, would you like to wash between your legs?' or if you were being jovial you'd hear people say 'I'll wash down as far as possible and you wash "possible"'. And all this sort of thing – how do you ask someone if they'd like to wash between their legs. . . . The language is **always** a problem.*

One of the major problems of language in nursing care is that there are no widely accepted standards for the names of body parts and functions. If, for instance, nurses call various body parts by their anatomical names, there is a fair chance the patient will not understand, and if they use language that is in common usage, the choice is by no means simple, and furthermore, there are some things which people do not readily discuss.

Yes, I do feel – I feel a bit of a jerk going up and saying – I don't say 'farted' [but] 'have you passed wind?' Yeah, I do get a little bit embarrassed that way. Funny you know, I can say 'have you had your bowels open?', that doesn't worry me, 'have you urinated' or whatever, that doesn't worry me but . . .

******

I think . . . [some] patients, when we ask them if they've had their bowels open, they tend to say 'yes' routinely because they don't know what we're talking about. That happens on a regular basis because they're not real sure what we're talking about. . . . People tend to call having your bowels open a lot of stupid things. . . . I think it's classed as dirty. Whereas it shouldn't be. It's only your own body, but I think they're taught from a young age [that it's dirty].

With the civilising process (Elias 1978), body functions concerned with excretion have become highly privatised, at least by some social groups, particularly those of higher social status. Waddington (1973:219) has argued also that there are class differences in the way the body was regarded during the civilising process and that these class differences extend to both linguistic and environmental privatisations. I was interested, therefore, to hear if nurses had perceptions of class difference in approaches to the body and body functions, especially in relation to talk about bodily functions. It would appear, at least from these accounts, that the arguments of Elias (1978) and Waddington (1973) about class difference in degrees of 'civilisation' are supported by the experiences of two nurses with respect to language and discussion of body functions.

*You were told all the correct terminology. If you didn't deviate off that it was O.K. Well it was easy to ask if they'd used a pan or a bottle, that was easy. When they asked 'what for?' it was difficult. (Laughter) If it was a bottle you were safe. I remember one little boy . . . and I asked him if he'd been to the toilet and he said 'what for?' So I said 'have you done a poo?' and I went through everything, and eventually I said 'have you shit today?' I had to! It was the only terminology. At times **you have to come down to their level** [emphasis added]. There is no way round it, especially if it's important.*

******

Oh yes. I think it's definitely class related. Joe Bloggs off the river bank is easy to talk to. They shit, they fart, they piss. You can communicate. It's the people with a middle-class presentation who don't have the vocabulary to match.

In summary, therefore, learning to be a nurse involves facing the reality of the place of the body in our society. For beginning nurses the body is the focal point for learning new behaviours typical of the occupation. Becoming socialised as a nurse, however, means taking on a new way of looking at the body and learning to 'do for'. It requires un-learning ways of viewing the body. Such un-learning is necessitated by 'the problem of the body' and by the extent to which nursing and illness are disruptive of social order and normal rules do not always apply. In Foucault's terms (see Chapter 2) nursing has the added problem of power/knowledge because there is limited discourse on the body and some of its functions. There is also no professional jargon that can be used to describe body functions which would make it possible to sanitise things people regard as dirty. Terms such as 'have you had your bowels open?' are the closest one can come to talking in a professional language, but there are people who do not know what that term means. In the absence of discourse and socially acceptable language, some nursing functions are located outside socially condoned and accepted practices – they are dealt with by their absence and the silence which surrounds them. They are actions which belong to a particular context of privatisation, at least in (some parts of) this culture. Because of the need to manage the body, nurses develop specific occupational strategies which help them and their patients live through periods of 'doing for'. These strategies are discussed in the following chapter.

6. Embarrassment, social rules and the context of body care

This chapter and the one which follows outline how nurses manage the bodies of others using a somological approach. This chapter illustrates the extent to which body care is located in context, how that context is constructed and managed, what the taken-for-granted rules are which sustain the processes of care, and how important and fundamental the notion of embarrassment is to a somological understanding of the body in nursing practice.

During illness people are confronted with what Parker (1988:10) called 'the boundedness of embodiment' such that their need for assistance with privatised body functions can be both embarrassing and unprecedented in adult life. It can also be a time when patients experience a loss of control over the body, and that loss of control can also become a source of embarrassment. In a society which has privatised the body and (some) bodily functions, embarrassment is a powerful means of social control. However, we know very little about the management of embarrassment in social situations generally, and almost nothing about its management in situations when people need assistance with body care. I will argue here that the concept of embarrassment is central to understanding how nurses manage the body – but embarrassment in a nursing sense is a much richer concept than that which is used in popular language in relation to 'normal' social life.

THE NATURE AND MEANING OF EMBARRASSMENT

Heath (1988:136–137) claims that embarrassment has received little attention within the behavioural sciences and that sociology, as a discipline, has largely ignored the subject of emotions, including embarrassment even though it is a fundamental feature of social life.

Embarrassment lies at the heart of the social organization of day-to-day conduct. It provides a personal constraint on the behaviour of the individual in society and a public response to actions and activities considered problematic or untoward. Embarrassment and its potential plays an important part of sustaining the individual's commitment to social organization, values and convention. It permeates everyday life and our dealings with others. It informs ordinary conduct and bounds the individual's behaviour in areas of social life that formal and institutionalized constraints do not reach (Heath 1988:137).

Many sources of embarrassment we experience in social life relate to the body, its attire, its functions, and our capacity to control bodily processes such as burping, crying and yawning. We are taught, through mechanisms which act to maintain social order, to control ourselves in public life and to control embarrassment, or the potential for embarrassment. The literature on embarrassment consists predominantly of works in which the ideas of Goffman (1955, 1956) and Gross and Stone (1964) have been influential. More recently there have been a number of experimental studies within a psychological framework (Modigliani 1968, 1971, Apsler 1975, Fink & Walker 1977, Buss et al 1979, Foss & Crenshaw 1978, Levin & Arluke 1982, MacDonald & Davies 1983, Petronio 1984, Edelmann et al 1984, Edelmann & Hampson, 1979, 1981a, 1981b, Edelmann 1985,). Many of these studies have been designed to test hypotheses derived, in part, from Goffman's theoretical work. There have been only two reports of work done outside experimental settings, those by Weinberg (1965, 1968) on nudist camps.

A number of features of embarrassment appear to have been established. It is an organised aspect of social life which is culturally and contextually influenced, and it is recognised by characteristic behavioural changes (Edelmann & Hampson, 1979, 1981b), of which facial expression and body movements, taken together, are the most accurate indicators (Edelmann & Hampson, 1981a). Capacity for embarrassment appears to develop at about the age of 5 years (Buss et al 1979), embarrassment requires an audience (see, in particular, MacDonald & Davies 1983), it is more acute if the audience consists of strangers (MacDonald & Davies 1983), and it is a process where rules are broken and mechanisms are employed to restore composure (Edelmann 1985). Males, it seems, use defensive strategies, while females use protective strategies (excuses and justifications) to regain composure (Petronio 1984). One study, which has important implications for nurses showed that compliance in social situations increases if the person is embarrassed (Apsler 1975).

Two research papers (Foss & Crenshaw 1978, Edelmann et al 1984) have claimed also that the likelihood of helping behaviour is reduced if a person is embarrassed. These two studies, however, use experimental conditions which limit the extent to which their claims can be accepted. Foss and Crenshaw (1978) used a 2 × 2 design for high or low embarrassment and dropped either a box of envelopes or a box of Tampax (tampons) in front of samples of men and women. There was a significantly lower incidence of the article being retrieved by the target person depending on what was dropped – fewer people picked up the Tampax. The design does not take into account, however, the actual and potential symbolic meanings attached to sanitary items associated with menstruation. There is more to be considered in their study than embarrassment alone, particularly taken-for-granted ideas and attitudes which concern the body in our society. The other study, by Edelmann et al (1984), is similarly flawed because they also used Tampax as part of their 2 × 2 design, contrasting it with a box of tea.

In 1981, Edelmann summarised the literature on embarrassment and clarified some conceptual aspects, including its definition. He reached several conclusions about what had been established at that time, and he proposed a psychological model for understanding it as an interpersonal and social process. He defines embarrassment as 'a common and often dramatic experience' consisting of 'a highly uncomfortable psychological state, which can have a severely disruptive effect on social interaction' (1981:125) because it 'can be attributed to the violation of social expectations which govern and define desirable behaviour' (1981:126). He also argues that embarrassment must be differentiated from shame because the former is possible only in the presence of a real or imagined audience and that it is, therefore, an interpersonal process, while the latter is a personal and private experience. That is not to say that the two cannot co-exist. However, 'the crucial condition necessary for embarrassment to occur is that an individual behaves in a manner inconsistent with the way in which he or she would have wished to behave' (Edelmann 1981:132).

There is a high level of consensus among those who have written on this topic that social rules are fundamental to embarrassment and that embarrassment occurs when rules are broken. However, embarrassment does not necessarily follow if the rule-breaker is unaware of the rules or deliberately chooses to break them (Edelmann 1981:132).

There are several problems with the research on embarrassment. The first problem is that the literature is predominantly psychological and experimental to the extent that, with the exception of Weinberg's (1965, 1968) work, embarrassment has been studied under contrived conditions, usually, but not always, involving public places. As one would expect of psychology, it has focused on the effects of embarrassing situations on individuals. Second, little work has been done on establishing the rules which define some things as embarrassing and others as not embarrassing. Why, for example, did the researchers choose to use Tampax as an item which could induce embarrassment? Third, these studies have all been conducted on healthy 'normal' people, and not people who are ill and for whom, therefore, there may be little scope to initiate socially restorative mechanisms.

Weinberg's studies of nudism

Weinberg's (1965, 1968) work, in contrast to the psychological studies, is useful for our purposes because it illustrates the rules that exist to govern the management of nudity. However, the setting is quite different, being among those who frequent nudist camps. He used participant observation, interviews and question-naire data to illustrate the importance of context in being a nudist. He found that nudists experienced no embarrassment while they were in the camp. However, the same nudism, he suggests, would be embarrassing at home. He found that a system of rules helps establish the context in which non-embarrassing nudism is possible.

Weinberg (1968) proposed a model that governs situations in which embarrassment could occur. His model has two dimensions: (1) the definition of the situation, which means how one interprets one's own actions or what one assumes to be the interpretations of others; and (2) the nature of the act, that is, if it was intended or unintended. A four-cell matrix is possible with this model so that there are four possible outcomes of any situation:

(1) An intended act carried out in a correctly defined situation does not result in embarrassment;

(2) An intended act which is carried out in an incorrectly defined situation is a potentially embarrassing *faux pas*. (The

example he gives is a situation where one dresses too casually for the occasion);

(3) An unintended act in a correctly defined situation is another potentially embarrassing situation – a *social mistake*; and

(4) An unintended act which is carried out in a situation that has been incorrectly defined. The eventuality here is an *accident*. (The example he gives here is a situation where a woman mistakenly, but not deliberately, walks on the beach without the top piece of her swimming costume.)

He also claims that if situations are incorrectly defined they may lead to unintended acts so that mistakes, faux pas, and accidents are not mutually exclusive. Presumably, however, as one becomes a nudist, or a nurse, or a patient, a transition period is necessary in which one learns the rules and definitions of situations. Outcome (1) above, for example, feels comfortable (and therefore not embarrassing) for the person only when that person has attached meaning to various acts and situations. The question of intentionality must also be considered. For instance, a person may know what the rules are but deliberately choose to break them.

What Weinberg and others who have studied embarrassment have not questioned is why the body and some of its functions are embarrassing nor do they tell us what processes give rise to the evolution of particular rules which sustain definitions of situations in which embarrassment can occur. There is no explanation from Weinberg (1968) why he chose to illustrate his model using the example of a woman who bared her breasts, just as there are no explanations from Foss and Crenshaw (1978) or Edelmann et al (1984) as to why a sanitary item associated with menstruation would induce embarrassment.

The civilised body and embarrassment in nursing

In a 'civilised' society, people cover their bodies and there are rules which govern the circumstances in which it is socially acceptable to be naked, or to be relatively naked. For example, examination of the body by a medical practitioner is an occasion when it is acceptable to expose the body (see Emerson 1971), but there are strict taken-for-granted rules which apply. In the circumstances which often prevail during hospitalisation, however, both patient and nurse must negotiate the process of 'handing over' (on the part of the patient) and 'taking over' (on the part of the nurses) the body for its physical care. Consequently, there are rules which normally apply in society to be considered, such as the expectation that people will show some modesty about body exposure, there are rules which make it acceptable for nurses to take other people's clothes off, wash their bodies and help them with toileting, and there are rules which govern the timing of the 'handing over'/ 'taking over' process. However, Weinberg's (1968) two organising factors, the definition of the situation and the intended or unintended nature of the act, mean that managing embarrassment can be problematic for the patient and the nurse.

Defining the situation correctly requires knowledge of what is expected and acceptable. Experienced patients know these rules but nurses constantly encounter patients who are experiencing their first episode of hospitalisation. What is more, because nurses 'do for' patients in private and out of public view, there is a limit to what a patient **can** know unless the patient has had previous experience with hospitalisation. In addition, while patients may have been taught that some bodily functions ought to be done in private, when they are hospitalised they may not be able to do this, and so they must re-define situations. There is an added difficulty when patients lose control of bodily functions and as a consequence they are embarrassed about unintended acts on their part – acts which in normal circumstances they could control.

In his 1965 paper, Weinberg outlined the rules which governed the construction of a context in which nudism was not subject to embarrassment. Staring was proscribed, as was sexually explicit talk or 'dirty' jokes, body contact (including dancing which was regarded as sexual), and alcohol consumption. Photography was also restricted. Additionally, nudists are expected to adopt a frame of reference to the body and body exposure which defines nudity as natural and normal. He noted also that this naturalistic approach to the body extended to bodily functions so that toilets were not gender-specific. He did not explain an apparent incongruity, however, in that the toilets had doors, albeit three-quarter length. Clearly nudists were not entirely naturalistic about those body functions which required toilets.

The rules that Weinberg's (1965) study identified have parallels in nursing. It is not considered appropriate in nursing, for example, to stare or to make any comments to a patient about their body other than that which is relevant to their condition or care, although nurses may share comments privately among colleagues. For example, they may tell colleagues about a particularly nice body with an all-over suntan. Anything which is sexually explicit in patient care is also heavily proscribed, and any encounter with a patient which involves exposure of the body takes place in a context which is constructed as a nursing environment and not something else, e.g. a sexual encounter. There is also the expectation that body products are part of normal physiology. It is a basic rule in nursing that unnecessary exposure of the body or nakedness is to be avoided because it interferes with 'privacy' (discussed in Chapter 7) and may embarrass the patient, or in the case of nurses' social mistakes it may embarrass the nurse.

It was on a night that we had a lot of [post-operative] cystoscopies, T.U.R.s ... and – I will never forget this night! There were two of us [nurses] and we went into the room and pulled down the patient's bedclothes and (laughter) – I will never forget – he was only young and what we realised after was that he'd had a meniscectomy (laughter) and he turned around and said 'My God, you're so thorough!' I walked out of that room and never went back in there again. Thank goodness he wasn't in [hospital] many days and, you know, we joked later. . . . But we went and just pulled down the entire covers and lifted the gown up! You know still to this day I don't know who was more shocked. He was smiling, we [nurses] were both devastated. You know it was incredible. I'll never forget that. (Laughter)

This account illustrates not only that context is a fragile thing but also that normal social rules do not cease to apply when one is hospitalised. It is only socially acceptable for nurses to have access to the body in keeping with the patient's condition. The nurses' embarrassment in the account above was not due to **what** had been done because clearly they had been inspecting the genitals of other male patients, but it broke the rules in being out of context for a nurse to inspect the genitals of a patient who had undergone knee surgery.

NURSES' DEFINITION AND MANAGEMENT OF EMBARRASSMENT

Fundamental to helping patients with their bodies during illness, with their situated dependence, is help to manage embarrassment. When it is applied to what they perceive patients experience, nurses use the term embarrassment in a richer and more global sense than the definition provided by Edelmann (1981), and it means more than rule-breaking (discussed in more detail in Chapter 7). Integral to nurses' construction of embarrassment are notions associated with the patient's vulnerability, dependence, and social discomfort and they regard embarrassment as a consequence of inadequate protection of the patient's 'privacy'. They also use embarrassment to describe how patients react when they are experiencing physical changes to their bodies. Before it is possible for nurses to help patients, they must first learn to manage their own embarrassment, but like so many other aspects of body care in nursing, this is not an explicit subject of instruction or education.

Nurses' management of their own embarrassment

The nurses I interviewed had no recollections of ever having been taught how they should manage their own embarrassment. What they knew they had learned from experience. It appears that, in most cases, the embarrassment they experience is often acute at the beginning of their careers but fades very quickly with practice. I heard many times that the first time they ever washed another person was the worst and most embarrassing experience as beginners, although there were exceptions. After the initial experience there seemed to be little difficulty with their own embarrassment unless a patient broke the rules that the nurse took for granted, particular if this involved a sexual definition of the situation. There are also, of course, situations such as the one outlined above, where nurses may make their own social mistakes, but they are fewer than those made by patients, and that is logical – nurses are in an environment where they are very familiar with the rules and patients may not be.

Managing embarrassment has an element of teaching and coaching whereby the nurse leads the patient in defining situations that may be novel for the patient. If nurses are not embarrassed, it gives permission for the patient also to feel no embarrassment, but nurses must firstly learn to manage their own embarrassment and to convey the impression that they are not feeling uncomfortable. Managing one's own embarrassment gets easier with experience and with age, although age does not necessarily bring less embarrassment. One of the interviewees, who worked for many years teaching student nurses, had observed that mature age students cope no better with embarrassment than their younger colleagues. The crucial element would appear to be experience. Experience not only brings greater skill, which enables the nurse to feel more technically competent, but it also brings a greater sense of confidence and knowledge, which make the situation more manageable.

There is another crucial element in the management of embarrassment, and that is the sense of purpose associated with having to perform particular nursing acts. If there is a purpose which is explicit and accepted, potentially embarrassing situations become manageable. One male registered nurse provided a very clear illustration of this sense of purpose.

[As a student] I was seconded to the [X] Hospital for Women . . . for 2 or 3 months and I was working in the ante-natal ward roaming around conducting breast checks for reasons that I was unsure. Now I found that situation highly embarrassing. . . . I had to check peri[neum]s and the whole lot, but it was the breasts that got me because I didn't know why the hell I was looking at them. (Laughter) I had to ask all these women all the time 'can I see your breasts?' and I must have been a bright shade of red . . . I think it made them feel embarrassed. After a few tortuous days . . . I finally sought to find out why I was looking at breasts, and [I found that] there were breast abscesses and cracked nipples and redness . . . . I could include a few aesthetics as well . . . but . . . I was certainly relieved to know why I was looking at breasts . . . . So long as I can establish a logical reason for being there and doing what I'm doing, then I can apply reason to my action and establish a logical . . . framework and do it. If the individual [patient] has a problem with me doing it then I can say 'look, this is why I'm doing it'.

There are particular methods that nurses use to manage their own embarrassment. They use speed as a way of minimising the time they are exposed to certain situations, although this tends to be a technique which they use less and less as they become more experienced. They also talk among their colleagues and share their experiences so that the collegial sense of understanding makes it manageable – if others have had similar experiences it becomes something inherent in the nature of their work and not a personal failing if they feel embarrassment. In this sense shared reality is manageable reality. Nurses also adopt a sort of fatalistic approach to these things that is summarised in their notion, 'it has to be done', which means they can define a situation as unavoidable. This notion is extremely common and I heard it many times, not only with respect to embarrassment, but also with reference to many things in nursing which are aesthetically unpleasant. The following account gives an indication of the constellation and integration of techniques nurses use to manage their own embarrassment, and it indicates how their approach to the patient involves the patient in defining a situation fatalistically – 'it has to be done' – and both the patient and the nurse share that perception.

I.   *[I'd use] various tactics. Laughter, jokes, wear a mask, total silence. Never anything rude, in laughing or joking. Verbally there wasn't any sort of seriousness, you know.*

R.   *Was it ever OK to make your embarrassment explicit, and say to someone 'I'm really embarrassed doing this'?*

I.   Yes, that would depend very much on the person [and] what you were
doing with them. If you had someone, say, who you'd struck up a bit of
rapport with, in those instances it became quite comfortable, and you'd
*think 'Oh God, I've gotta do this **again**' and in you'd travel with your*
trolley, you bag of goodies or whatever and say [to the patient] 'look
love, here we go again!'.

If the patient is not perceived by the nurse to be embarrassed, then
it is very likely the nurse will also feel little embarrassment – there
will be a reciprocity of perspective that makes the situation much
easier to manage for both patient and nurse.

I think they [patients] can make you or break you. . . . You get a person who
understands the situation and they make it very easy for you and then again
you get someone . . . [who gets embarrassed very easily] – they make it jolly
hard.

Nurses' perceptions of what indicates embarrassment are central to
how they approach the patient, how they feel themselves, and how
the encounter with the patient will be managed. Recognition of the
potential for embarrassment is, however, fundamental to viewing
the encounter in context and viewing it somologically. If the patient's
embarrassment is an issue for the nurse when nursing care involves
'invading' the patient's body, there is a mutual recognition of the
embodied experience of the patient. Non-recognition of potential
embarrassment for the patient, on the other hand, reduces the
patient to an object.

Recognising patients' embarrassment

The literature suggest that there are well recognised behaviours
which indicate embarrassment, some of which are universal in
humans, such as blushing, and some are culturally defined.
Edelmann and Hampson (1979, 1981a, 1981b) have established
that embarrassment is indicated by reduced eye contact, increased
body movement, smiling, and changes in speech patterns, and Fink
and Walker (1977) have noted that humour is often also used.
   I asked the interviewees what they perceived to be indicators of
embarrassment in patients. They confirmed each of Edelmann and
Hampson's (1979, 1981a, 1981b) indicators, and also that humour
was often used among colleagues. Humour is almost a standard
way of coping, but it is used judiciously with patients, and the
notions, 'it depends on the patient' and 'it depends on the situation'
govern its use. Patients who are in need of nursing care are often
not in a state where laughter is possible or appropriate, so this
makes sense. People with abdominal wounds, for example, find it

painful to laugh, and there are some situations where laughter would be completely inappropriate. In their use of humour nurses take their cues from what they know about patients' personalities, and sometimes it is the patients who indicate that humour is a way of managing some things, in which case it is relatively easy for the nurse to share in that humour. There are other indicators nurses interpret as meaning that the patient is embarrassed.

They [patients] go red, they get sweaty or giggly, or they keep saying they're sorry . . . or keep apologising.

★★★★★★

[Patients will] change the subject. Usually turn red, they look uncomfortable, fidget, pull the covers up, avoid the situation altogether.

★★★★★★

They might hedge around . . . .

★★★★★★

Some people just tell you.

★★★★★★

They sort of wrap their arms up a bit, around themselves and hang on to the sheets or whatever, put it round themselves, firmly. Sitting up in chairs they will cover urine bags – things like that – hide them.

★★★★★★

They hide. They tend to cover themselves very quickly. Sometimes they will say things like 'I'll do it, I'll do it, it's alright'. Sometimes they can and sometimes they can't.

As in most things related to nursing care, knowledge of the patient is important and the perception of embarrassment is based, in part, on that knowledge of how the patient behaves in other situations. Both the following accounts illustrate the importance of locating individual patient behaviour in the context of that patient's established way of responding.

Obviously there are clear things like blushing . . . but I don't think blushing is as common as looking at the ceiling and excessive chatter, on the other hand extreme silence for some that may talk a lot anyway – to be suddenly very quiet, and turn away. I think they're the best indicators for me, but that comes from knowing the patient as well . . . .

★★★★★★

If they've established a normal repertoire of behaviours and they don't adhere to that repertoire of behaviours. The obvious signs of embarrassment that you would recognise are changes in facial colour, tendency not to maintain eye contact, general signs of introversion . . . . I think there's also an aggressive demonstration of embarrassment too, and probably a depressive demonstration of embarrassment.

Sometimes there are very subtle changes in the way patients respond which are interpreted as embarrassment. For example, one midwife, as well as illustrating the need to know the patient 'in the situation', contrasted how a patient's responses to two different nursing procedures indicates embarrassment. One situation requires access to the patients arm – a 'safe' area to touch (Jourard 1966, 1967, Jourard & Rubin 1968) and the other procedure is vaginal examination during labour.

It depends. And it is hard if you have never come across this particular patient before. But if you've worked with the patient doing non-embarrassing things then just the change in their tone, their attitude, their body language or – again it's how long you've known the person. It's little things other people mightn't notice because they all give signs that they're embarrassed. They don't all go red, or pull the sheet up over their head. They all give signs that they are embarrassed. . . . You will go in there [to the patient] and say 'I'm going to take your blood pressure' she'll stick our her arm, but if you go in there and say 'I've got to examine you' and instead of quickly getting themselves organised their movements are a little slower . . . – facial expression may not change all that much, but just enough to notice.

From the point of view of illness experience, many things which nurses do with and for patients, and many of the things which patients do when the nurse is present, break rules that would ordinarily apply in society. However, by the way they manage their own responses and by their lack of embarrassment (affect), nurses re-define situations for patients so that the patient need not feel embarrassed. It is a way of indicating to the patient that it is permissible to vomit in front of someone else, and to have someone help them with defaecation. It is a way of showing the patient that a situation is manageable. It is also a way of indicating to the patient that the body and body functions, irrespective of how privatised they are normally, can be integrated into experience.

BODY CARE FOR OTHERS AND FOUR BASIC SOMOLOGICAL RULES

In the context of hospitalisation, people will let nurses do things to them and with them that would be impossible and unthinkable for many in 'normal' social life. People in hospital are amazingly compliant with nurses' requests and give nurses permission to have the sort of intimate contact with their bodies that many have never experienced before, and which many will never again experience except during subsequent hospitalisations. The data reported in this chapter attempt to address specifically the context in which patients need assistance with what Turner (1984:1) called 'the details of corporeal existence', and the rules which help construct and sustain that context.

Several important interrelated factors operate to form a system of basic rules which nurses learn from practice and which they expect the patient to respect, and there are also specific contextors which nurses need to use in order to create a nursing environment. Some of these rules appear self-evident and obvious, but they nevertheless need to be made explicit because they form part of the taken-for-granted social environment in which nursing is practised – a kind of social ecology to the extent that they form a system. The rules are: (1) the compliance and control rule, (2) the dependency rule, (3) the modesty rule, and (4) the protection rule. The first three rules are illustrated well by drawing on the concept of the 'good patient' while the protection rule is discussed in detail in the next chapter.

The good patient and basic rules in the context of nursing

Central to a 'good' working relationship between the nurse and the patient is an understanding that patients are expected to comply with what the nurse wants them to do and that the patient does not resist or obstruct the nurse. The nurse assumes and at times demands control. 'Good' patients relinquish that control and unpopular patients do not (Taylor 1979, Lorber 1975, Bhanumathi 1977, Kelly 1982, Stockwell 1984). The research data reported in this book indicated that the compliance and control rule follows a pattern which corresponds to trajectories of recovery or dying (discussed in detail in Chapter 8), and that the nurse has a certain definition of what makes a 'good' patient depending on where that patient is on a trajectory. I was not surprised, therefore, to hear that nurses expected patients to be co-operative if not compliant because all the literature suggest this to be so. This is what two of the registered nurses said patients did to help the nurse.

Co-operate. (Laughter) Do what you want . . . . I guess they make it easier if they let you get on and do what you want to do, get it over and done with.

******

Just being helpful, not lying there like a log, so to speak, . . . [and being] alert to what the nurse is doing and assist.

There are, however, some subtle, and also some very overt, aspects of what the nurse regards as compliance that were highlighted in the accounts I recorded. Nurses recognise that the patient is at a social disadvantage, that the nurse has a more powerful position than the patient, and that the compliance patients display is due in part to that power differential.

Basically, nurses have an incredible amount of power . . . [over patients]. Most of them don't realise that. They are very powerful people. You get somebody who is an executive or up-market business person, or anybody – doesn't matter who they are – come into hospital and all of a sudden they're subservient, you know. No matter who they are. It's the way you treat them. You bring them into hospital, strip them of all their clothes, put them in pyjamas and shove them in bed and tell them to behave. And people take it!

There are times during a patient's hospitalisation when the only functional arrangement between the nurse and the patient is for the patient to be completely (or almost completely) dependent on the nurse for body care. This is the dependency rule, and it is particularly obvious when the patient is so ill or sedated that it is physically impossible to do otherwise (this is discussed in more detail in Chapter 8 in relation to recovery). Such dependence does not mean, as one nurse put it, that the patient should lie in bed 'like a beached whale' and expect the nurse to literally do everything.

The modesty rule is closely related to the other three rules and it means that the patient is expected to be neither too modest or embarrassed, nor too free to expose himself or herself, and that the nurse will protect the patient's privacy. The following two accounts illustrate, in particular, what this rule means and how it interrelates with the other three rules. In effect the patient is expected to let the nurse have control and to comply with the nurses' requests, to be appropriately modest, and for their part, nurses acknowledge a need for protection of patients – it is a reciprocal arrangement.

R. *What makes a 'good' patient?*
I. *Ones that will let you do anything. (Laughter) No. I expect the patient to try and do things for themselves and you expect them to be a bit modest but they're in hospital and you've got to do these things for them so you expect them to let you do the things, whereas some patients won't let you near them, but you do expect – you just expect them to act like a patient! (Laughter) . . . . Somebody sick in bed and you're caring for them so they should just let you do your duties.*
R. *They should let the nurse take control?*

I.   *Yes. That's what you expect. I suppose we shouldn't really, because it's their own body and they should be in control of that.*

******

I.   *A 'good' patient will make it easy for you by just chatting and not feeling embarrassed, they roll over when you tell them to roll over, they don't splash water all over the place. These are silly little things – interrupt the cycle by wanting to use a bedpan in the middle of a sponge, not questioning you a little too much.*

R.   *So you expect the patient to be docile?*

I.   *Oh yes! . . . That's a sad outlook, because I think that's when you get to know the people you're looking after the best, when you're invading their personal space like that, and that's when you need to be the most careful about what you say and almost not alarming them about anything.*

The modesty rule is of particular relevance when nurses undress and expose patient's bodies, handle them and wash them – experiences which the patient may be having for the first time. Again there is an expectation that the patient is co-operative, and they are expected to show some modesty but not so much that they are 'too embarrassed' because they then become difficult for the nurse to manage. Patients who are very embarrassed at having their bodies exposed create their own particular kind of problems.

Some people are just so embarrassed, they've got their arms across their chest the whole time. You've got to prise them back and wash them. . . . Some people are just so shy and embarrassed – I think for the older [patients] that it was all taboo to be uncovered in front of anybody.

******

It's difficult if the patients are so embarrassed they don't want you to do it, but they're not capable of doing it themselves either, you know, physically incapable of doing it themselves. . . . And they're clutching and [saying] 'it's alright, it's just been done', and you know it hasn't.

Patients who are not embarrassed but who appear quite relaxed are, by comparison, much easier for nurses to manage, though this is not always the case. Nearly all the problems which the interviewees identified with respect to this rule concerned sexually explicit or sexually suggestive behaviour on the part of the patient. This is behaviour which is inappropriate to nurses' definition of the situation, and it breaks the rule which governs their ideas about modesty and embarrassment. It seems that nurses expect that patients should show some embarrassment during body care, and those who do not can be perceived to be breaking the rules.

I think this turns every midwife off – the lady who has the see-through nighties – and you can see her pads. . . . It looks absolutely disgusting. It's terrible to see a lady waddling down the corridor with a view of everything. It offends a lot of people. It doesn't offend me, I just think 'oh, no!'

******

You might try to keep their modesty or whatever ... keeping them covered . . . and they might rip it all off and just sit there and [you say] 'cover yourself up'. . . . You might have them covered over and the sheet might slip off as though it's an accident (laughter) and you just cover them over again . . . – they're a flasher.

Sexual expression as rule breaking

In body care specifically, then, behaviour which breaks the rule about modesty challenges the nurse's definitions of situations, and it is perceived by nurses as sexual. Generally, this type of behaviour fits into two categories. First, there is the unwarranted and unnecessary exposure of those parts of the body which people would usually keep covered in public. Such behaviour may be accompanied by sexual suggestion to the nurse. Second, there is inappropriate defining of a situation as a sexual event. Both of these types of behaviour require social management, and may be defined by the nurse as a form of sexual harassment (discussed in detail in Chapter 9). They are useful episodes to examine because, as examples of rule breaking, they help identify what is assumed by the nurse about the body and how it can be managed socially.

I suppose . . . the ideal expected way is for everyone to be proper . . . [but] it doesn't always work that way. . . . When you do sense that somebody's having a great time [inappropriately gaining sexual pleasure from nursing care] you tend to get a bit hot under the collar and think 'damn you, . . . you're enjoying everything that's happening. I'm not'. And there is an acceptable way [for patients to behave during nursing care] and once it gets a bit beyond that and into the stage of their [sexual] pleasure, well, yes, you do tend to get a bit . . . (Laughter). . . . You get an incident whereby a patient really enjoys a scrotal shave – it's very hard because you tend to – you don't quite know how to cope – as you get older it gets a bit easier . . . .

Sexually explicit behaviour on the part of the patient which results from their defining the situation differently from the nurse is especially difficult because there is no shared reality. The nurse defines the situation as a nursing encounter and the patient has something sexual in mind. It is also possible that, for some patients, there is no difference between a nursing experience and a sexual experience – they are one in the same thing.

The patient has to – the patient has to play the role or they can make you terribly embarrassed. . . . For instance, I had to put some vaginal pessaries into an old lady. Now the accepted role for the old lady would be for her to lie back, put her legs in the position I asked her to, allow me to do it without making it physically difficult, and generally talk about something other than what I was doing, other than perhaps to make a comment like 'that's uncomfortable' or something necessary to the procedure. This old lady, when I put the pessary in said 'oh, give me a bit of dick', and I was utterly mortified! Because that's unacceptable behaviour, you don't bring a pleasurable, sexual connotation into it.

******

The ones that make it really hard for you are the . . . types . . . [who] like to show they can get erections and all sorts of things while you're sponging them . . . . They're the ones that make it difficult.

A common theme which underlies each of the accounts mentioned so far in this chapter is the importance of the context in which basic nursing care (body care) takes place. It is a context which the nurse needs to construct but which is simultaneously relatively fragile and easily undone. Nurses negotiate the socially delicate territory of invading another person's space in intimate ways by using specific methods, which they employ within careful social boundaries associated with the patient's level of dependence and illness. They follow the taken-for-granted rules which have been outlined here, and they also draw on occupationally specific methods which help manage such events. These methods are individual contextors which, taken in combination and depending on the situation, create a social environment in which acts of nursing care concerning the body are possible.

CONTEXTORS FOR NURSING PRACTICE

There are five main contextors which I identified which contribute to the structuring of situations as nursing practice. Two of these centre on the persona of the nurse (the uniform and 'the manner') and the other three (minifism, asking relatives and visitors to leave, and discourse privatisations) are deliberate nursing acts which confer a protective and private social atmosphere on the situation. The uniform and the manner are discussed here, and the other three methods are discussed in the next chapter.

The nurse's uniform

The nurse's uniform is fundamental and many believe it is essential in making nursing acts permissible, not only because of what the uniform symbolises to the patient, but also because it can be part of the nurse's identity without which practice would be more difficult (if not impossible for some).

I think probably the uniform is almost paramount because if that same person came in [to the patient's room] without a uniform on, and with a dish [of water] she might get away with it if the patient knew that person to be a nurse, but if that patient didn't know that person to be a nurse, then he would have no yardstick to allow it. I believe the uniform is paramount.

For some the uniform not only provides an essential element (contextor) in a nursing encounter but it also helps the nurse. It becomes part or the image, the persona, the identity, and many do not feel they are 'in the role', as it were, unless that uniform is there. And some use it as a form of protection.

I.   *I know one thing for sure, that when you put on the uniform you're taking on a lot more than just a job. There's something that goes with it. Some people give you more respect. . . . I suppose some people use their uniform as a barrier too.*
R.   *Protection?*
I.   *Protection, yes.*
R.   *Could you do what you have to do without your uniform?*
I.   *No. Definitely not!*

*****

I.   *Oh, no! [I couldn't cope without my uniform.] Take that off and that would be . . . a different situation. (Laughter) I wouldn't be too sure what I was doing! No, I'm sure it [the uniform] does [protect you]. You know, I think you – you take that away from – you hide a fair bit behind your title, you know. If you're a nurse, that's great. I guess that gives you the right to do all these things to people.*
R.   *You say you're a nurse and people drop their pants and?*
I.   *Yeah, well that's right! (Laughter) 'Don't worry about her, she's seen it all'. So you do. You do hide behind it [the uniform]. If you took that [uniform] away and you went to approach people on these sorts of things you'd be locked up, you know – you've got to hide behind it.*

Another registered nurse saw the function of the uniform in terms of the meaning it conferred on the role of the nurse and on the sort of things nurses do for patients. Because so much of what nurses do is intimately related to the body, and because the body is heavily inscribed with sexual meaning (particularly when it concerns the sort of body care that nurses do) there is a need to eliminate the sexual element of this intimacy. She explained it this way:

I think it's possibly tied up with sexuality, that if you put all nurses in the same uniform, without ear-rings, without jewellery, without make-up, without any of the trappings that make them traditionally sexual creatures, you can then – it's a bit like the grandmother in the rocking chair. You can stereotype this person, de-sexualise them, and they can then do those things in a nursing context.

The manner

The uniform alone, however, is not sufficient to bestow a nursing context on an encounter with a patient, there is also what could be called 'the manner' – a particular style of personal presence that is variously described as 'being professional', 'being clinical', 'being matter-of-fact', 'appearing as though you know what you're doing', 'being in control', 'appearing as though you have done this a million times before'. All of these are an affect that nurses were taught early in their careers.

I.   *It's a job . . . and it has to be done, and . . . if you go at it confidently and do not appear embarrassed, then your patient won't be embarrassed.*
R.   *So part of learning how to do it is to do it with a sense of what you could call – for want of a better term – a 'professional' air about you.*
I.   *Yes.*

The registered nurse who provided this account had worked in a variety of clinical settings including critical care and acute care areas, in the community, and district nursing where she did body care for people in their own homes. She was able to draw some clear distinctions between providing care for people in hospital and doing that same thing in people's homes. Without the confines of the hospital the encounter is vastly different. The patient has much greater control at home.

The atmosphere itself is certainly different, because you're on their turf now, so it's their home, it's their shower, so they sort of call the shots. They say 'I want this done, I want this like that', you know. . . . The whole environment changes for you.

The manner of the nurse, while it is part of a sense of personal competence that one needs to do these things, also relates to acknowledging the potential for the patient to become embarrassed or compromised in some way by what the nurse does. It is also very effective at minimising a felt sense of vulnerability. Much of the work of context construction that nurses do, including the use of a particular manner, is overtly concerned with protecting the patient's vulnerability and privacy.

In summary, nurses' work involves establishing social order when patients' everyday lives are disrupted. Nurses must deliberately construct a context which allows the body and the embarrassment associated with exposure, dependence, and illness to be managed in a particular occupational context – a context where the definition of the situation is not necessarily shared by patients. The definition of situations as nursing care rely on a set of rules that are learned through practice, and which may or may not be known (or adhered to) by patients. Those rules govern the management of the body and embarrassment during body care. They are social rules which are necessary in a society where the body and (some) body functions have been privatised and such rules are also used in order to make nursing practice socially permissible.

7. The body, illness experience and nursing

This chapter describes how nurses relate to patients and how that relationship takes account of certain key facets of illness. The discussion and the data show how nurses can help people through the experience of illness and dependency, particularly with a somological approach to practice. Nurses learn from experience that during illness the mind and body are emotionally, intellectually and practically inseparable, but that in the context of living through illness, some people cope with their bodies by objectifying or disowning the part which is affected. They also learn that despite the aesthetically unpleasant and potentially nauseating things that occur during illness, the patient is also a person, and that by their manner (among other things) nurses help patients cope with the body and what ails it. This illustrates how the protection rule is put into action. All of these things are made possible by the development of a relationship which is specific to the context of nursing, by the use of specific techniques, and by an approach to the body which allows nurses to practise somologically.

THE RELATIONSHIP BETWEEN PATIENT AND NURSE

Nurses understand how the relationship between the nurse and patient is crucial in illness experience. Expert nurses understand it very well (Benner & Wrubel 1988) and the data reported here come predominantly from experts. Such data therefore illustrate how nursing can be practised at its best and the data are not necessarily typical of nurses generally. Nurses understand, though, irrespective of their status as experts (or non-experts) that the patient is not just a body, but at times some 'get through' a particular procedure by focusing on the routine of the procedure. Nursing care, therefore, takes place in the context of the acknowledged personhood of the other. One of the interviewees put it very plainly indeed.

If you're looking after a person . . . then you're looking after them as a person and bodily functions are part of being a person . . . .

When nurses who are experienced and expert at their work 'look after' people, they do so in a way that considers the personality and particular circumstances of individual patients. The notions 'it depends on the person' and 'it depends on the situation' apply here as they do for so much other nursing care. Benner and Wrubel have described how

the best nursing practitioners . . . seek the patient's story in formal and informal nursing histories, because they know every illness has a story – plans are threatened or thwarted, relationships are disturbed, and symptoms become laden with meaning depending on what else is happening in the person's life. Understanding the meaning of the illness can facilitate treatment and cure. Even when no treatment is available and no cure is possible, understanding the meaning of the illness for the person and for that person's life is a form of healing, in that such understanding can overcome the sense of alienation, loss of self-understanding, and loss of social integration that accompany illness (1988:9).

The relationship that a nurse has with a hospitalised patient is context related and situational. It is unlike a 'normal' social relationship because it is formed during a time when the patient is undergoing what Newman (1984) has described as one of the most stressful personal experiences in technological society. In acute care settings it is a relationship based on mutual recognition of two things – the patient's vulnerability, and the patient's partial or complete dependence on the nurse for help with events which, in their everyday lives, people do for themselves. In the context of hospitalisation and in a situation of needing assistance with body care, tasks which are usually simple can become complicated – tasks such as going to the toilet, showering, and cleaning your teeth.

Normally nurse-patient relationships have a clear beginning, a course or trajectory, and an end. Nurse-patient relationships are also time related because, as the patient's hospitalisation progresses, the degree of dependence on the nurse varies and the relationship is re-negotiated on the basis of that level of dependence (discussed in the next chapter). Nurses also know that patients are vulnerable, that they are in unfamiliar surroundings, and that they may know little of what lies ahead for them. Nurses understand that particular patients may be facing an uncertain or unwanted diagnosis, or that they may be ignorant of what hospitalisation means for them.

Recognition of patients' vulnerability

Two interviewees described how they perceived the situation of the patient in hospital.

People [patients] are very susceptible to the likes of us because it's the only situation they're in whereby you are back to the 'grass roots' level so to speak. . . . That's a very vulnerable situation for people to be in, I mean they're reliant on you in most ways and for everything . . . I don't think people quite realise just how vulnerable they are, or they're going to be.

******

As a nurse you get very intimate – not only physically intimate [with patients]. You're catching somebody while they really are down . . . – I guess you could say some nurses believe they're seeing people at their very base, the very element of their –. . . . You see them at their most vulnerable. I don't necessarily agree that you're seeing them at their plainest, or their true selves. Nevertheless, you are seeing them at their most vulnerable . . .

My field notes for the time when I was hospitalised make special mention of my feelings of vulnerability. In my case I knew very well what to expect with respect to the events which were to take place, but on the day of admission to hospital I had written that I felt a 'sense of vulnerability' which came mostly from a diffuse fear about unknown persons in whom I would have to place a great deal of trust. And it was also a fear about my own responses to what lay ahead. Would I be a 'good patient'? Would I be difficult to look after? Would I be embarrassed when my body was exposed to strangers?

My notes also record that this sense of vulnerability 'quickly fades on encounter with staff'. The process of establishing relationships with nursing staff developed very quickly and I recorded several key aspects of it. I was aware of Benner's (1982a:407) claim that nurses can create a context of acceptance for patients by their approach, particularly to wounds and by 'the way they talk of recovery'.

In the context of my admission, however, I was struck by the speed and apparent ease by which the nurses' approach made my sense of vulnerability manageable. Firstly, they were very skilled in their use of humour and they coupled it with a lack of surprise at a few aspects of my medical history which I knew to be unusual. Secondly, I had noted that a lack of surprise – almost lack of affect

– in the nurses' behaviour created what I call an *environment of permission*. This environment of permission is a social construct – an end result of the manner and approach of the staff. In many ways it is a construct which gives some control to the patient, at least in so far as it indicates to the patient a sense that everything is normal, that it is alright to feel anxious and vulnerable and uncomfortable in unfamiliar surroundings. In many ways, I experienced what Benner (1982a:407) had described as a 'context of acceptance', but in this instance the approach was used to make a particular phase of the patient experience manageable. My experience, however, is to be seen in the context of a routine admission to a private hospital. I also was not admitted for any condition which would be perceived as self inflicted or the result of a deviant lifestyle – a situation which may have contributed to a different reception.

The hospitalised patient is surrounded by nurses who are comfortable and familiar with the environment and by going about their work as 'business as usual' they set the scene for the patient. I had noticed aspects of this during my first field experience, but I found it particularly salient when I was part of the process and it was my own personal experience that I was recording. In creating this environment of permission, the nurses who were assigned to me very skillfully used a number of methods to define the situation, so that actions which would otherwise be most unusual were seen as very ordinary and unremarkable.

In this chapter, data from the interviews illustrate in much more detail what that environment of permission means to nurses, and how they deliberately construct it. Fundamental to this process is the recognition that the patient feels vulnerable, that the patient's 'privacy' needs to be considered, and that the relationship the nurse has with the patient is constructed on these assumptions. I asked the interviewees what methods they use to help them with the management of nursing care when patients felt vulnerable and when intimate contact with the body occurs. Their responses reveal highly complex considerations which are not easily reduced to a simpler level of understanding. Nonetheless, I was able to identify salient aspects of their practice. In doing that I do not wish to create the impression that such a reductive approach indicates that nursing practice can be reduced to component parts. My task is to build an understanding of the somological way nurses practise and I want to identify the social methods they employed to manage situations when they violate taken-for-granted rules about the body in society.

The nurse-patient relationship and the body

The people I interviewed had great difficulty articulating exactly what they did that helped them manage body care for patients. One of them remarked in exasperation 'gosh, it's hard to put into words and the questions are so simple'. So much of their skill and the way they approach patients is taken for granted, and for some things there is no language to describe what they want to say. It was at this point that I specifically used Garfinkel's (1967) notion of examining what happens when social rules are broken by asking them if they had ever had to nurse someone they knew socially and what problems, if any, that created. I was aware that on this topic I was asking them to talk about their own perceived shortcomings.

R.   *Do you find it more difficult or less difficult to look after people you know?*

I.   *More difficult until you can break the ice with what you say. I had a friend in here [as a patient] recently and I found it harder to sponge him, and I kept on talking, prattling on possibly. I found it hard to wash [him] and when it came time to wash the genitals I was lucky, he could do it for himself. But it is embarrassing.*

R.   *Is that because you have an established relationship?*

I.   *And it doesn't include nakedness.*

R.   *And it doesn't include doing for them what they normally do for themselves?*

I.   *That's right. Your association with them has nothing to do with their bodies.*

R.   *So you then have to step into almost an entirely different situation?*

I.   *Yes, and forget about – the rules for what you had before just do not apply, the association and relationship that you have is still there but you have to step into this area that's been ignored up till then.*

R.   *And you have to associate with them again socially afterwards.*

I.   *Yes. You do forget it. I do.*

R.   *What do you think about in situations like that where you are breaking the [rules of the] social relationship that you had?*

I.   *I think of their embarrassment more than anything. I felt embarrassed for him because I realised that he is not an exhibitionist, he is a very modest man, and I felt embarrassed for him more than myself because I had to do for men a million times before. I can switch off and do a routine sponge, but to that man it was not at all routine.*

For various reasons some nurses find it difficult to nurse people they knew, some found it made little difference, and others found it a very satisfying experience. It depended, however, on three things – the kind of pre-existing relationship that the nurse and the patient had, the patient, and the patient's particular condition. Some nurses described how everyday social relationships differ from those which the nurse develops with a patient. If nurse and patient have an established social relationship, new ways of relating to each other may need to be established because the previous social relationship does not extend to the things the nurse has to do in caring for that person.

I.   *You sort of – like you want to give them special treatment, and you do feel more uncomfortable with their private parts. . . . It's because you know them personally. . . . Because you know them, you're meeting them every day and . . . . . . It does depend on the person. And the fact that the person knows that you're going to be seeing them in a situation where they are unable to do anything for themselves. They might feel self-conscious about the fact that they were in that position. . . . And you feel it too. It depends how you go about it and what sort of social relationship you have with them.*

R.   *It does mean that you have to change that relationship if you have to do for them as a nurse.*

I.   *Modify it, yes.*

These accounts illustrate the context specific nature of the relationship of the nurse to the patient when patients need body care, but there are other ways in which a pre-existing relationship may interfere with nurses' abilities to function as they would with strangers. The account related below illustrates not only that the nurse-patient relationship is often one of sharing the patient's lived body experience, but also how a pre-existing relationship gets in the way, as it were, of relating as nurse and patient. It also shows how the object body (or what has happened to it) as well as the person has to be considered by the nurse.

[It was] awful. Just awful. It was [X] when she first had Crohn's disease. She went to theatre expecting to have part of her large bowel removed and came back with an ileostomy which . . . was mooted to be a permanent ileostomy. That was very difficult. I was on night duty and she was in the ward where I was working. And that was very difficult. . . . She says now it was good that I was there. . . . I find the difficulty [is] in dealing with someone's emotions, in that when she started to cry I cried too. I lost all grasp of what had happened and I fell into her category of 'it's unfair, why me' ra, ra, ra. . . . – I lost it all for about an hour and a half. She went through all the bits about it being unfair and "I wish I was dead", "I can't live with this", and "how will it be when I get home?" and all this sort of carry on, which are all quite reasonable . . . but I lost all grasp. Had it been someone I didn't know I may well have been able to make some sort of appropriate

responses . . . and I wouldn't have been lost in that emotional circle because
we were friends. . . . I could do all those things like sponge her and that, and
I think I probably took more care and was far better with her than with
anyone else, but I think the emotional thing. I don't think she was
embarrassed that I was washing her, I think she was too sick to care anyway,
and it was good that it was someone that she knew. But I think it was the
emotional thing, the illness that she had and the major surgery that she had.

It is impossible to summarise easily what transpires between a
nurse and a patient, because it is such a complex social phenomenon,
and it varies with each individual encounter. What is clear from the
accounts above, is that the social climate of the nurse-patient
relationship is a special kind of relationship – a relationship in
which the nurse needs access to ways of behaving which sustain
professional conduct and which help perform care for individual
patients. It is a relationship which must be established and
constructed on taken-for-granted premises about what the nurse
and patient roles imply.

Without exception my interviewees told me that the status of the
patient made little if any difference to body care, and they gave
examples of having nursed former Prime Ministers, politicians,
rock stars and other public figures. The only concern they expressed
was that the patient was sometimes in a position to complain about
the care they received, or to register disapproval, but where body
care was concerned the interviewees made comments like 'you've
seen so many naked bodies and this one was no different'. The
status of the patient seemed, therefore, to have little impact on the
nurses' approach to the body and body care, though they confessed
to being more wary because of the patient's potential influence.

The relationship the patient and nurse share with respect to body
care is difficult to describe or illustrate, but it is possible to get a
progressively more comprehensive picture of this relationship by
examining the ways in which nurses help patients with their bodies
in illness experience – how they use somology in practice.

THE SOMOLOGICAL APPROACH IN PRACTICE

When nurses practise somologically they not only take account of
the physical body (a thing) and the body as it is experienced, lived,
and felt by the patient but they also integrate these two aspects of
human embodiment. For example, if we take a scenario where a
patient has a gangrenous foot and is therefore also systemically ill
from the toxicity of the gangrene, in simple terms the nurse can do

one of three things: (1) practise objectively and reductively by focusing attention on the obvious signs and symptoms, document them and compare them with previous observations in order to arrive at a judgement about progress – all of which can be done sympathetically and kindly, but the primary attention is directed at pathology; (2) concentrate on the patient's lived experience and attend to the feelings associated with the problem and provide medication to relieve headache and nausea, leaving to others (medical practitioners) the problem of pathology; or (3) practise in a way which integrates the pathological problem of a gangrenous foot into lived experience so that the patient's situation is seen compositely. In crude terms this can be expressed as: (1) How is your foot (asking about physical symptoms)?, (2) How do you feel (asking about feelings which are not necessarily physical)?; or (3) Do you still feel sick now that you've had a look at your foot (integrating the body as object with the body as it is experienced)?

In effect, therefore, nurses who practise somologically are not only concerned with the body as an object and its associated social symbolism, they are also concerned with what we call the lived body in illness experience. They use a number of strategies to support somological practice so that the body in illness experience is perceived as manageable. Such methods are often direct, overt and specific to particular patients or conditions. They rely heavily on trust and the confidence of the individual nurse and they are probably best understood as abilities of expert nurses (see Benner 1984) because they require a high level of clinical skill and sometimes courage. Some examples drawn from the interview data illustrate this type of practice clearly.

Examples of somological practice

In the following account, which was related by an experienced and expert midwife, I had asked how she behaved toward a woman who had had a truly awful experience in labour, or who had delivered a stillborn baby?

Um, I think personally, I don't care if I cry in front of them, it sometimes helps if they know that if whoever is doing it – well, she's a person after all. I think it helps, you know, if you get tears in your eyes and what have you, it gives them permission to cry in front of you . . . But, I mean, you give your feelings. Like cleft palates and cleft lips. And . . . you've got to allow them to say 'yeah, it looks terrible, it looks horrible' [and to say to them] 'I know why you're upset and it's alright to be upset, it's alright not to like how your baby looks'. That's just because I've been here for a while. . . . I think that just

*takes time – to come across these things and you have to have personal
contact, you can't learn it out of the book . . . and sort yourself out about how
you react and you would feel if it was your baby. And when you know
yourself it makes it easier for you to understand other people's feelings.*

This account not only illustrates that experience informs the ways
in which nurses practise, but also how honesty can be used to
establish reciprocity of perspective with a patient, to share a common
reality and trust. Without a common reality and trust there is little
basis for an on-going relationship, and that relationship is essential
if the nurse is to help a patient. These features are also illustrated
in the account below, and in addition it illustrates how a subtle use
of time and encouragement bordering on challenge can function as
a method to help patients with their bodies, especially if they have
been disfigured. This account outlines somological practice in the
management of a change in body image, and where attention to the
visual impact of that change is thought to be therapeutic for the
patient. It is a commonly held belief among nurses that before
people can come to a resolution of what has happened with their
bodies, patients must first look at what has changed.

I.   *People don't like ugliness. It's like when you take a mastectomy dressing
      down for the first time.*
R.   *They [patients] won't look at it.*
I.   *No.*
R.   *How do you get them to look at it?*
I.   *There's no other way than to tell them that the mirror is there and when
      they're ready, have a good look. Sometimes people like you to be with
      them when they do it and others, you know, they like you to leave them
      and in their own time they do it. . . . If they say 'this is awful', then you
      have to agree with it. You couldn't say 'no it's not' . . .*
R.   *Is that part . . . of developing a sense of trust with the patient?*
I.   *Oh, they couldn't trust you if you weren't honest.*

Sometimes encouragement bordering on challenge can proceed to
pressure leading to confrontation, especially if the patient seems to
be a little too slow from the nurse's point of view about how long
these things should take (but that will be discussed in relation to
the recovery trajectory which is described in the next chapter).
However, such pressure would come only if more subtle methods
failed. The sense of shared reality between the nurse and the
patient begins to break down when the nurse sees something as
manageable and the patient does not see the same possibility.
Ostomy patients are particularly good examples through which to
illustrate the sense of inability to cope. Nurses often use the term
'embarrassment' to describe this sort of inability to cope with the

body, and this is one illustration of how a term in common usage has a particular meaning in nursing. In this nursing sense 'embarrassment' means that a patient has not integrated object reality (say a change in the body) with existential reality (what it feels like to visualise a changed body). The following account illustrates this use of the term 'embarrassment' as well as the nurse's understanding of the patient's body as it is experienced.

I.   *A colostomy is a very difficult thing to deal with. If the patient is not able to cope with it [clean it] themselves, they are usually highly embarrassed at you having to do that for them. . . . With a colostomy you're facing them.*

R.   *Is it the colostomy as a thing or their embarrassment and emotional response that's the difficult thing?*

I.   *They don't like you having to look after them when they've had their colostomy opened. They just don't like it. Usually.*

R.   *Why is that, do you think?*

I.   *I guess that is society, you know, when you have your bowels open you do go behind a closed door and that's it. Here they are, sitting up there large as life and you've got to do that for them. And they are embarrassed. . . . They don't like it being there anyway. They just don't like owning it . . . as though it's something they'd like to chop off.*

In situations like that outlined above nurses will use a number of methods. They will show the patient by their actions when they clean a colostomy that it does not nauseate the nurse, that they have done the same procedure 'a million times before'. They may tell the patient that, yes, they wouldn't like it if the same thing happened to them, but they will also coach the patient and teach them how to manage it. And if the patient chooses to give the colostomy a name (such as 'Henry') and distance themselves from it, nurses may go along with the naming, or alternatively make no comment. If the patient chooses to cope in that way, they will be allowed to do so, and nurses may become part of sharing the patient's methods and take it for granted that some people cope that way. The following account outlines that well. I had asked this registered nurse, who had considerable experience in a range of fields, if she had ever seen patients objectify a part of their body, for example by calling their diseased foot, **the** foot, instead of **my** foot.

*I didn't take any notice of that . . . because they're probably trying to dissociate it from the body aren't they. If they're calling it **the** instead of **mine**. They don't want it as theirs, they don't want that part of them. I don't know if I've ever looked at it quite as blatantly as that before. I nursed all those years and I haven't thought much about it.*

This last account illustrates the difficulty of researching nursing practice because, not only is it highly complex, it must also be understood as a social process and learning to practise nursing requires the nurse to develop ways of managing the body as a biological and social entity, not only as it affects the patient, but also as it affects the nurse. These are best illustrated by examining how nurses deal with the interface between the biological and the social aspects of being. Nurses must simultaneously practise in a way which takes account of 'the problem of the body' in civilised society, the biological aspects of being (for example, excretion) and they must do so in a way which recognises the vulnerability and dependence of patients and how they feel themselves. All of these things can be understood as facets of the protection rule (mentioned in Chapter 6).

THE PROTECTION RULE IN NURSING PRACTICE

During my first period of field observation I noted that nurses were protective of the patient, and some seemed to almost assume a sense of ownership of the patient. Protection acknowledges patients' potential for feeling embarrassed in needing help or being unable to maintain total control of the body or ensuring their own privacy for body functions. For example, some people do not like anyone present if they need to vomit.

Sometimes nurses also protect their patients from visitors and relatives, and sometimes sending the relatives and visitors away protects the nurse. In fact, many of the protective things that nurses do assist both patient and nurse by functioning to make the body, and some aspects of nursing care, private. Such protective methods are also for patients' 'privacy' – again this is a quite different notion from the common meaning of privacy, that is, withdrawing from public or being out of the public arena.

Protecting the patients' privacy

The notion of 'privacy', as nurses use it, is difficult to articulate. It is related to a recognition that some bodily functions are attended to without others present. Bates (1964:431) claims that 'there is general acceptance of the notion that a person should be accorded privacy in a number of ways with respect to the body and its functions' and that 'this can be seen not only in the matter of bodily exposure, but in relation to waste elimination'.

However, for nurses in this study, 'privacy' is at the same time both very concrete and abstract. It means all of the following, either individually or in combination – a lack of audience, no unnecessary exposure of the body, minimising the possibility of embarrassment (as one would commonly use the term – not in its nursing sense), maintaining a person's dignity, and an aspect of personhood. Respecting 'privacy' is a fundamental principle of practice, and much of what nurses do when they help patients with the body is done in the context of the need to protect 'privacy', among other things. 'Privacy' is an underlying assumption on which the protection rule is based, but the need for protection goes beyond the patients' need for 'privacy' by assisting nurses in the management of what they do for patients.

I have called one of the methods they use *minifisms* – techniques whereby the nurse deliberately and overtly understates the situation or minimises the extent of something. Another way of ensuring protection is by reducing the audience in one of two ways – asking relatives and visitors to leave and what I call *discourse privatisations*. This 'need' for the relatives to leave is sometimes fabricated by the nurse as a plausible excuse to ask visitors to leave so the patient can get some rest but mostly it is used when the nurse tends the patient for body care. Discourse privatisations mean that the nurse uses a form of discourse with the patient which ensures that certain body functions and aspects of patient care are discussed as a private matter between the nurse and the patient. These strategies not only protect patients from feeling subject to normal social rules, they also reduce the extent of potential embarrassment, and they minimise the patient's feelings of vulnerability and loss of 'privacy'.

Minifisms

Minifisms can be verbal and/or behavioural techniques which assist in the management of potentially problematic situations by minimising the size, significance, or severity of an event involving a patient. They are also methods of bringing a situation under control. From observation I noted such techniques appeared to 'come naturally' in nursing encounters with patients. In order to probe this behaviour I devised a technique at interview where I outlined a small scenario and asked the interviewees if they had witnessed what I described and why they thought nurses responded as they did. My typical question was:

Have you ever seen a situation where nurses will minimise or trivialise or understate something? Say, for example, a patient has vomited all over the *bed and made a terrible mess and the nurse will say to the patient, 'you've made a **bit** of a mess'?*

All but a couple of the very inexperienced nurses knew exactly what I meant and many of them laughed when I outlined the scenario and we discussed it. One gave me a very graphic illustration of what I was talking about.

I.   *'Don't worry about it. It'll be alright'. [The nurse says.]*
R.   *Yes, 'you've made a bit of a mess'.*
I.   *(Laughter) Yes.*
R.   *Or bled all over the place and the nurse says 'you've had a bit of a bleed'.*
I.   *Yes 'don't worry about it'. But can I just take you along a bit further. . . . You'll do that in front of the patient but then you'll go out the back ... and say 'fuck', you know, 'look at **this**'. Or ... 'come here [X] has just – you've gotta help me, he's just – **all over the place**' and you go in [to the patient's room] and you're almost patronising once you get to the patient.*
R.   *And you tell the patient you do this every day. 'It's perfectly alright'.*
I.   *Yeah.*

The reasons why the interviewees thought nurses did these things vary a little but all reasons essentially have something to do with the notion that the nurse needs to create an accepting social situation for the patient – that *environment of permission* mentioned earlier. Their explanations centred on the idea that the nurse's role is to make the situation acceptable for the patient and that in some ways it helps nurses not to dwell so heavily on the situation that they lose their composure. Minifisms are used to manage the patient's embarrassment and help the nurse to behave as though everything is 'business-as-usual' – one aspect of the approach they use to create an environment of permission. Although minifisms are probably a more generalised social phenomenon than I have indicated here, they are particularly advantageous in nursing situations. The accounts illustrate their use and the extent to which they assume that the nurse's role involves protecting the patient and patients' potentially negative perceptions and feelings.

It's obviously an embarrassment for the person you're looking after – they're gonna feel embarrassed, they know they've made a rotten mess, you know they've made a rotten mess. So you say 'that's O.K., no problem' ... Yes. You know how they feel awful. I know I do it all the time, [say to the patient] 'it's O.K.'.

Some nurses see minifisms as methods which limit any distress the patient may feel and as a way of not exacerbating a situation. Minifisms are a way of controlling what has happened and they prevent the situation from deteriorating for the patient. By using minifisms they can define that situation as unremarkable.

Oh yes, you see that a lot (Laughter). They [nurses] do [use minifisms]! They do that because they don't want to alarm the patient. I mean . . . if you're the nurse and you're standing at the end of the bed and say 'you've had a little sick-up' the patient's not going to think it's a great worry are they. They're gonna think 'she doesn't think it's much so maybe it just looks more than it is'. . . . But I've seen them [nurses] go the other way too. Panic. Does nothing for the patient! (Laughter)

*****

By not really letting the patient know that they have been horribly sick – are they trying to protect the patient – 'that's not really 2 pints of blood on the floor there'. (Laughter) They're sort of reassuring the patient in their own back-handed way and maybe they're covering up their own [feelings by saying] 'my God, I've got to mop it all up', 'she missed the bowl again' (Laughter).

Minifisms apply in the context of patients' inability to avoid a situation and when physiological processes (or pathological processes) render it impossible for them to have control over what is happening. If, however, patients have a level of control and could possibly have avoided the mess, in the nurse's perception, then nurses may not use minifisms. The two following accounts illustrate the difference in the nurse's approach if the patient is believed to be in some way responsible for making a mess unnecessarily.

I. I guess . . . you try to keep the patient from becoming upset . . . [and it] does help you [also]. You don't want to make a fuss about it, it's part of your job anyway and they [patients] feel as though they're putting a big strain on you. . . .

R. So if you understate it, it makes it O.K. for the patient?

I. It makes it more O.K., it's never O.K. for the patient. And . . . this is part of my job, I don't mind doing it, it's just something that happens. . . .

R. But nurses are not as forgiving if the patient has control are they?

I. No, if they vomit all over the bedclothes and they have a vomit bowl there, you tend to get a bit hard to that person.

******

I. Yes, I think it's for . . . patient protection. I think . . . people feel embarrassed – the dependency on people to do things for them that they would normally do – . . . an invasion of privacy . . . they feel bad enough anyway that they've made this mess and someone has to clean it up. But to walk in and say 'uh, . . . look at the bloody mess!' will make them feel twice as bad. And I think nurses trivialise that sort of thing . . . to ease the patient's anxiety about dependency and that sort of thing.

. . . But then while nurses trivialise in front of the patient they will often walk outside the room and complain and swear.
R.   *'Wouldn't you think he could have hit the dish'.*
I.   *Yes, or 'why did she have to miss the pan?'*

Nurses often use humour as an aspect of minifisms and in conjunction with other methods to help each other manage situations from the viewpoint of their own feelings and sometimes to protect the feelings of the patient. However, humour is not always available to the nurse because the context can be inappropriate. Some of the interviewees in this study see minifisms as a nursing-specific way for them to use humour, especially if it helps them manage their own embarrassment because it is one way of restoring composure and it can be used as an alternative to embarrassment (see Fink & Walker 1977).

It's your own way of keeping your humour. Well if you lose that you wouldn't cope. . . . I think sometimes our humour to others is perhaps a bit of a sick one, but then it's your only way to cope with what you have to do. You boil underneath with those sort of situations – having things [body products, usually faeces] rubbed up against bed-rails and all the rest of it. I mean – it doesn't matter where you touch, if you don't laugh well, what would you do? You'd walk away. You'd never come back. So I guess in a way we do, we say things to minimise the embarrassment of the patient but in actual fact when you look at it – No! It's probably just to keep yourself on an even keel and handle it.

Like other aspects of nursing practice, minifisms not only understate the dimensions of some problems nurses deal with, they can also operate to render care invisible, and they can therefore contribute to its being poorly valued. If nurses themselves do not overtly acknowledge the real nature of their work and the extent to which it requires, like other types of women's work, considerable emotional labour (see Hochschild 1983), they have a double bind. To make their true feelings felt would clearly not be in the patients' interests, but not to do so contributes to the camouflaging and privatising of nursing work. In fact, one of the problems of nurses' work in a 'civilised' society is that in order to protect patients' 'privacy' they deliberately reduce the audience by asking relatives and visitors to leave.

Asking relatives and visitors to leave

When nurses assist patients with body care they will usually ask relatives and visitors to leave the room. This is one method by which they protect the patient's 'privacy'. It is a firmly established and traditional practice of nurses, although it is no longer applied as a blanket rule in all situations. It now tends to vary according to the patient and the nature of the relationship of the patient to the relatives and visitors. Many of the people I interviewed could remember being taught that relatives and visitors always vacated the patient's room (or vicinity) during nursing procedures. It was a standard and invariable rule, but not many could remember the precise purpose for which it was intended other than that it was a means of protecting the patient's 'privacy'.

I.   *I think it is changing. We never did any sort of procedure on a patient with relatives [present] then [prior to the 1970s], but then the relatives went out for any reason. Like if the doctor came, they were sent outside. Whatever you did, they were sent outside, they were just not there.*

R.   *Why was that? It was a very consistent practice.*

I.   *Oh absolutely! You never did anything with a person standing by. I can't even remember the reason given. . . . Perhaps part of it was the embarrassment for the patient . . . revealing any part of the body. I think part of it also was that the nurse didn't want to be watched. . . . It was just a general thing, the thing was between the patient and the nurse and no-one else had any right to be there, not even his spouse.*

R.   *So why wouldn't a nurse want anyone watching?*

I.   *I think it was just the done thing, that they weren't there.*

R.   *Is it sometimes that the nurse finds whatever she had to do for people difficult and the smaller the audience the better?*

I.   *I'm sure that's part of it for some things, yes.*

As well as considering the patient's 'privacy', sending relatives and visitors out of the room is also a method by which nurses: (1) minimise their own potential embarrassment; (2) manage their dirty work by having it hidden from view; and (3) feel less exposed to potential criticism or interference from relatives and visitors. At times it is also necessary for nurses to be aware that some relatives and visitors do not have the personal fortitude to watch some things that nurses do, or that they may become upset by witnessing the suffering of their loved ones. In essence, having access to the patient's body and performing body care for the patient is easier if there is no audience – there is a smaller potential for embarrassment either on the part of the nurse or the patient. The two accounts below summarise these functions.

It depends on what relationship there is. Usually if it's a husband or next of kin it's alright to let them stay. It's becoming more prevalent to let the husband stay [in midwifery in particular], but if it's children, or aunties, or sisters . . . some of the procedures that we do will expose certain parts of that patient that perhaps they mightn't feel comfortable exposing to that relative.

And often with injections a lot of people are upset by those things anyway. I think that tends to be the reasons that we sent them out. The other thing is that they don't interfere with what you're doing because you get some [who will interfere].

******

I think they're sent away for various reasons. I think they're sent away to help the nurse manage embarrassment, . . . if you are a bit insecure and you don't want people to see maybe you won't do whatever you're doing perfectly. If they're not there then it doesn't matter if you take some short cuts, and also I think that nurses have traditionally felt that relatives can't cope with unusual or invasive or embarrassing things being done to the patient and so you manage it by putting them outside. If they're not watching they don't know what's going on and you can go back out and say 'Dad's comfortable now' and they haven't watched you perhaps put this poor old guy through agony as you turned him or they haven't seen the big hole in his backside that you've been dressing. And so you're able to hide a lot from the relatives. . . . Part of it is to protect the relatives and I think certainly a lot of it is to protect the nurse from various things.

Asking relatives and visitors to leave is also one method of managing what Strauss (1987:122–123) has called 'wife work' and 'attendant work' that takes place when a husband is hospitalised because there is confusion over the boundaries of the wife and attendant (nurse) roles. The boundaries are blurred because the wife may be used to doing certain things for her husband but in the context of the hospital the attendant (nurse) is also used to doing those same things for patients. Strauss has seen it as an exclusive phenomenon where the wife is shut out of a caring role for her husband. The experience of two people I interviewed seems to indicate, however, that the phenomenon Strauss identified exists beyond the husband and wife relationship. Their accounts are related below.

Last year when Mum was in hospital . . . I was not permitted, although . . . everyone knew I was a registered nurse, . . . to get her out of bed and walk her to the toilet.

******

My Dad's in hospital at the moment and I don't think anything of cleaning him up, but it's interesting [that] the nurses who work there don't think I should do it because he's my father. They get annoyed because I want to do things for him and they say 'no, no, we'll do it' . . . [especially when it concerns bodily functions like toileting].

Strauss' (1987:122–123) notion of the exclusive nature of wife work and attendant work does not fit with the accounts which I recorded for this research either. While there was widespread recognition that nurses are taught to do body care for the patient without the presence of relatives and visitors, it is not the exclusive process that he suggested. Many nurses now see it as appropriate for some relatives to assist in the care of their hospitalised family members, but again, there is considerable variation and the notions, 'it depends on the patient' and 'it depends on the situation', apply. That is, from the nurse's perspective, these things are managed in their context, although special status can still be given to some body functions.

I.   It's possibly – depending on who the visitors are for a start. . . . I think if one just had their neighbour popping in to bring you a bunch of flowers you wouldn't want them there while you had your dressing changed. So, um, there's that aspect of it. Also the visitor may not want to stay either. They may – might be all they can do to get themselves through the doors of the hospital and visit their member of the family let alone stay and look while you did the dressing, or give them a pan, or whatever. I can't say I've given that a great deal of thought. I know sometimes . . . that . . . if it's a husband – we tend to clarify who the visitors are – and ask if they **would** like to sometimes help, maybe, ... It depends on the circumstances.

R.   Is there more family participation in the care of patients than there used to be?

I.   Yes, I think so. I think particularly . . . with the longer term . . . terminal patients. We do encourage families to stay and if they want to wash their [relative's] hands and face, or feed them or do whatever for them, we don't discourage that, we do in fact . . . encourage it. But the other things – the dressings, pans, and things like that – probably they're private acts – going to the toilet and things like that – you don't pee with an audience so we ask people to [leave the room].

As well as protecting the patient's 'privacy' by asking people to leave the vicinity of the patient, linguistic methods can also be used.

Discourse privatisation

Nurses usually ensure that conversations about 'civilised' (privatised) body functions are restricted to the nurse and the patient by a method which I call *discourse privatisation*. Discourse privatisation is a function of the problem of language outlined in Chapter 5. This form of discourse not only protects patients' 'privacy' but it also protects nurses from potential embarrassment, except in cases where, for example, the patient is partially deaf or nurses must run through a repertoire of terms until they hit upon one the patient recognises. Discourse privatisation assists nurses in creating a particular context in which the patient relates to the nurse, and tells the nurse things about various body functions which would not normally be a subject of social conversation in 'civilised' society.

There are two basic conversational methods of using this technique: talking only to the patient in a low voice; or talking with the patient in spatial isolation so the potential hearing audience is restricted. The latter method means waiting till visitors have left or asking relatives to leave while the conversation is conducted, or by calling (mobile) patients aside and talking to them where others cannot hear. I had noted this technique during my field work and had it confirmed many times in my conversations with the interviewees. From their perspective, it is a necessary condition for maintaining the patient's 'privacy' because it bestows a privacy on what the nurse and the patient discuss.

This form of discourse with the patient could also be called a 'contextor' in the sense that it contributes to the creation of a particular context and reality based on the privatising of some bodily functions. In conjunction with the other strategies outlined here, discourse privatisation is an indication of how nursing practice must take account of biological and social factors where the body is concerned. It also illustrates that nurses integrate those factors into the everyday experiences of hospitalised patients in keeping with their somological approach in caring for others and in keeping with the protection rule. This is also clearly apparent in the ways nurses deal with situations which are nauseating and when they deal with body products.

Managing nauseating situations and body products

Chapter 2 noted that there are symbolic systems which govern approaches to body products and that, generally, there are social rules which govern body functions and body products. Because nurses have so much to do with body products, I wanted to know what particular body products were difficult to manage and why and also how they actually managed body products socially. There were no surprises here for me in relation to what they found difficult because I have worked as a registered nurse and I still practise, but nurses found two products most difficult to manage – faeces and sputum. Faeces is difficult to manage because of its smell and because sometimes patients are incontinent. In this respect, these nurses showed a similar regard for faeces as the medical students did in the Ross et al (1968) study (where medical students rated faeces as relatively dirty).

Why sputum should be so difficult is to some extent a mystery, but simply talking about it was nauseating enough for some, and they asked to change the subject. The only obvious answer would appear to lie in the fact that nurses must sometimes deal with large quantities of it from patients who have what is called a 'productive cough', and the sound of the cough is experienced as nauseating by some. Nurses are required, however, to make visual and written observations of the quantity, colour, consistency and sometimes the smell of sputum and things that smell are particularly difficult to manage. There appears also to be something about the slimy consistency of sputum that makes it aesthetically and practically difficult to manage. Knapp (1967:587) has suggested that humans have an innate sense of avoidance of things which feel slimy.

While I did not specifically seek information on the relative aesthetics of various body products, the data I collected would not support the Kubie (1937) model described in Chapter 2. Some of the people in my study found no particular body product problematic, rather, these products were accepted fatalistically as an aspect of nurses' work and the notion, 'you just have to do it' (a variation of 'it has to be done') became relevant.

The methods used by nurses, however, to deal with situations and products which are aesthetically unpleasant or nauseating, are varied, and they all take, as a fundamental rule, the belief that patients should be protected from perceptions that nurses find this sort of task difficult, and the nurse should not, therefore, exacerbate the situation for the patient by displaying any sense of discomfort. In practice this means never indicating to the patient that the nurse finds a particular task repulsive or nauseating – it is a form of emotional control consistent with Hochschild's (1983) notion of emotional labour. If, however, the task is unmistakeably aesthetically difficult, the nurse may use *minifisms* as a means of defining the situation as manageable, or honest and open talk to acknowledge that something is unpleasant, but this will be conveyed to the patient in a minifying context.

When they must do nauseating or aesthetically unpleasant tasks, nurses use a number of methods which are essentially intellectual exercises or psychological strategies to focus their attention on the mechanical and procedural aspects of the task, or they think of other things. They also take time out. Time out is invoked when something is particular difficult to endure, and the nurse makes some plausible excuse to the patient, such as, 'I have to go and get some more dressings' and then spends time outside the room regaining composure, especially with situations where the odour is oppressive. One registered nurse summarised his psychological strategies in this way.

I usually . . . psych up. . . . While I'm actually doing it I try to separate what I'm doing – make it a clinical function. And then afterwards, if I'm gonna be sick, that's when I'm sick.

Some of the interviewees, however, managed by deliberately focusing their attention on the experience of the patient and they use empathy, especially if they have to manage a wound dressing. The following two accounts, were given by very experienced nurses who have practised for many years with surgical patients where one is most likely to encounter difficult and smelly wounds. They both illustrate the perceived need to manage one's own responses as a way of making situations manageable for patients.

I. *I think that's very hard. I think for me personally I go back to feeling for the person, and your feelings are not so much for the things you've got to do, you have to revert and think if that's hard for us what's it like for the person –*

R. *So you would focus on the person and try to identify with that person.*

I. *Yes, I wouldn't say that you don't feel sick in the stomach, each time you have to deal with someone [nauseating]. . . .*

R. *Especially if is smells.*

I. *Yes, that's the hardest part. You can cope with anything unless its got the smell. That's where you're actually tending to want to heave each time you're going to tend to the person, but I still say it's alright for us. We have to do it, fine, but we can leave. You've gotta feel for that person who's with it [the smell] all the time.*

******

I. *I guess I'm thinking 'what a terrible mess', 'what a disfigurement', or 'what a terrible position to be in' – for the person to have to have this done . . . – faecal fistulas, radiation-type situations which can be terrible. That's the sort of thing when I think 'how awful to land up like this. Wouldn't it be awful to be this person'.*

R. *So you would identify with the person?*

I. *I think that's what I do. . . . I think that's how I cope. I think I do do that. . . . Sometimes it's mixed with anger if I think it's been somebody's fault, neglect, or –*

R. *Botched?*

I. *Botched, yes. And I get a strong angry feeling, which I try and hide. Nothing can be done [surgically or medically to repair the damage]. It's too late.*

R. *Do you hide your own emotions when you have to do things which are truly dreadful?*

I. *Yes, I think I do. When they're physical things like that. But I have long since given away the no-shame-of-the-grieving type emotion. Yes, I*

do hold myself very much in check with physical things. . . . I fully
subscribe to the fact that you hide the horribleness of it from the patient.

In adopting the approaches which have been described in this chapter and the previous chapter, nurses structure environments and define situations in ways that make it possible for patients to live through difficult and problematic experiences with illness, and with the sometimes horrible things that happen to bodies.

Nurses create an *environment of permission* for the patient in which to reconcile what has happened to their bodies, and that is made possible by the construction of a particular kind of relationship and by the use of clinical strategies which assist both the nurse and the patient. It is also made possible by the generalised context of hospitalisation, illness and dependence, as well as a number of occupationally specific strategies which nurses use to make nursing care possible. Such an approach is not always successful, but it creates a climate in which reconciliation and integration of the object body and lived experience of the body is possible, irrespective of whether the patient is going to recover or die.

The central notion which emerges from these data is that nurses practise in a way which takes account of the biological aspects of being and integrates them into lived and social experiences. Furthermore, this is done in a social context which acknowledges that the body is treated in particular ways in 'civilised' society and that some body functions are a source of potential embarrassment to people. What I call somology is characteristic of nursing practice in that the person and the body are viewed as an integrated composite, and part of nursing practice involves the facilitation of that integration. The patient is not just a body or body part, although that view is adopted in the short term to manage difficult situations. As an organising framework for knowledge derived from practice, anything less than an integrated and composite view, such as somology, will lead to a fragmentation of our understanding of embodied existence. There are also assumed rules which govern the processes by which such integration takes place in nursing, which nurses take for granted, particularly as they concern control of the body. This is illustrated further in the following chapter.

8. The body in recovery, dying and death

Most patients who are dependent on nurses during hospitalisation are either recovering from an acute health problem or they are going to die. Some patients may be hospitalised for a chronic condition from which recovery is not possible, but the nurse may still expect some recovery, even if it is only symptomatic. There are also patients for whom the outcome is uncertain, but such uncertainty is usually transitory.

This chapter illustrates how the compliance and control rule, and the protection rule, influence the ways in which the body and control over it are 'handed over' (by the patient) to the nurse (and 'taken over' by the nurse) during illness and dying and 'handed back'/'taken back' in recovery. It is also about the ways nurses perceive and manage death and the dead body, and the dependence the patient has on the nurse, how that dependence centres on what the patient cannot do without assistance and how it is negotiated between patient and nurse. Dependence, however, is a commonly used term and it has multiple meanings, some of them pejorative.

DEPENDENCE ON THE NURSE

Dependence is a state of reliance on something or someone and it takes many forms, but the one I am concerned with here is a short term, situationally defined dependence on another person, a nurse, for assistance in looking after one's own body care and body needs.

Patient dependency has been studied consistently in relation to health care for many years, mostly from a managerial perspective, in an attempt to establish accurate measures of how many nurses are required to provide care for patients with various conditions. Miller's (1984) review of the research literature on patient dependence suggests, however, that the study of patient dependency is problematic. She argues that nurses induce dependence in patients by reinforcing dependent behaviour; that they underestimate what a patient is capable of doing without assistance; and that this is particularly so where elderly patients are concerned. There are, however, few studies which deal with nurses' perceptions of what dependency means, and it is usually nurses who make decisions about dependency needs for individual patients.

What I am concerned with here is a quite different notion of dependency – the specific and temporary situational dependence that the nurse and patient negotiate when the patient needs short term assistance with body care.

Situated dependence and nurses' expectations

In the period of field work when I was a visitor, I noted that nurses had a very task-specific approach to what they regarded as situations when patients needed assistance. For example, they will do some things for patients and not others, and this seems to be based on what they define patients are capable of doing for themselves. It is not a generalised state, which seems to be the case when nurses deal exclusively with the elderly (see Miller 1984, Barton et al 1980).

During my period of hospitalisation, I asked some of the registered nurses about this task-specific approach to dependency that I had observed. One confirmed that nurses sometimes 'get pissed off with patients who go to the shower on their own, and then expect you to clean their teeth for them'. Similarly, another said that nurses also do not like patients who are capable of looking after themselves but who lie in bed expecting to be waited on as though the nurse was a servant.

I had also noted that nurses' expectations change over time as the patient recovers from illness or surgery, and that different activities are associated with different expectations, for example cleaning one's teeth, compared with getting in and out of bed. Dependence is thought of as a continuum which relates to temporal aspects of recovery or dying, although there are some things for which the nurse retains responsibility, such as the patient's bed and room. Some nurses also maintain a liaison and advocacy role for patients in dealing with other personnel, especially medical practitioners. This continuum has a pattern which can be described as a trajectory.

The recovery trajectory

These research data show that there is a recovery trajectory similar to the dying trajectory which Glaser and Strauss (1968:Ch. 1) described. The dying trajectory has two organising features – duration and shape (in that it can be graphed). Additionally, the perception of these properties depends on other perceptions and expectations of the pattern a particular patient will follow towards death (Glaser & Strauss 1968:6). It is patient specific in time and shape. Glaser and Strauss (1968:6–7) also identified 'critical junctures' – changes in the patient's condition for which nurses use physical indicators and the rate of decline as cues to the patient's location on the trajectory.

The Glaser and Strauss (1968) study, however, relied heavily on what they could observe nurses doing – a methodological approach which has subsequently been shown to be inadequate where nursing is concerned (see Lublin 1984). They also have a medico-dominant approach to nurses, which means that they tended to see (almost) all nursing actions as functions dependent on doctoring. Webster (1985) has shown, however, that the medical viewpoint is not very accurate about what nursing involves. Despite its shortcomings, the Glaser and Strauss (1968) study provides some very useful information about dying and nurses' perceptions of patients' expected progress, which could be used as a basis for describing the nature of the recovery trajectory and how it differs from, or is similar to, the dying trajectory.

RECOVERING, DYING AND HANDING OVER THE BODY

The recovery and dying trajectories have many features in common. They both have time and shape, they are marked by turning points – 'critical junctures' in dying and what I call 'recovery indicators' (because they occur for both improvement and setbacks) – and the trajectories are accompanied by expectations of a particular outcome – dying or recovery. Further, the dying trajectory is based on the belief that a patient will certainly die, and the recovery trajectory is based on the belief that the patient will recover. While these beliefs about the certainty of dying or recovering may seem self-evident, such beliefs are crucial to how nurses behave because they set up expectations and define a situation as either a dying or a recovery situation.

There are, however, subtle differences in the recovery and dying trajectories, and they pivot on who controls the patient's activities about body care, and who decides what bodily functions are 'handed over' and when they are 'handed over'.

Control, handing over and taking over the body

When the patient is believed to be capable of recovery, nurses maintain control over what the patient is expected to do, and the patient is expected to comply with those expectations — this represents the compliance and control rule in action. The dying patient, however, has more scope for making those decisions and this is usually done in consultation with nurses. In practice a great deal of consultation and negotiation takes place between nurses and patients in both situations, but what differs is that nurses will assert more pressure on the recovering patient to be mobile and resume responsibility for body care. They will encourage patients to be willing to have the body 'handed back' in order that they comply with the expected recovery trajectory. Dying patients, though, will be treated differently. They are allowed to determine more of their own level of dependence while also generally being encouraged by nurses to retain as much control as possible for as long as possible. That is, nurses try to delay, for as long as possible, the process whereby the patient 'hands over' and nurses 'take over' the body, but there is a tendency for (some) nurses to 'do for' the patient and in this way they encourage dependence.

Most of the time if we think they are not going to get better we won't worry so much about mobility . . ., like [we] don't make the patient sit out of bed for meals. You can ask them, but if they don't want to they don't. You don't push them.

Where recovery is expected there is the assumption, on the nurses' part, that the patient wants to recover and go home, yet in practice some patients like to be in hospital and attempt to find ways to stay there.

Some patients just think this is a holiday. They love the attention and have got no-where else to go – abuse the system. . . .

The recovery trajectory follows a pattern and timetable which is predominantly set by the nurse rather than the patient. Variations from this pattern, on the patient's part, may result in nurses re-interpreting their expectations of the patient's condition or being firmer in dealing with the patient. They sometimes also tell the patient that they are taking 'too long' to resume their normal activities. This is different from the reactions of nurses to patients who take longer than expected to die, or who die more rapidly than expected. The nurse will make plain to recovering patients what is expected of them when they do not follow the perceived normal recovery trajectory, but they will not behave similarly with the dying – they are more (publicly) tolerant of deviations from an expected dying trajectory.

Alternatively, patients who take 'too long' to recover may result in the nurse becoming extra vigilant about the possibility of complications and pressure on the patient to follow the normal trajectory may be reduced or it may cease.

I suppose the approach to the patient changes [if they are not fitting the nurse's expectations] and make it known to the patient that they should be doing more. . . . There's a hell of a lot of whingeing and bitching outside the room [among nurses] but it becomes, in a way, taboo to go and tell the patient 'you're just being lazy, get out of bed'. I think there's a lot more encouragement and pushing goes on, quite firmly. . . .

Just as there are patients who are 'too slow' to recover, there are those who recover too quickly for nurses' expectations. Such patients put the protection rule under strain by wanting to do things for themselves when their physiological condition is such that assistance is necessary.

The patient who wants to take themselves to the shower the day after an appendicectomy, or gets out of bed to use a bottle . . . [is] just as bad as someone who hangs around for three extra days and doesn't want to go home.

Situations where patients recover 'too quickly' not only strain the protection rule, they also illustrate somological practice because the nurse must deal with patients in a way which integrates patients' experience and wishes, existentially, with the more practical aspects of embodiment and the object body. For example, a patient may want to get out of bed, but the nurse takes account of the patient's condition. Irrespective of a patient's intentions and motivations, there are physiological (biological) considerations which will determine what is possible. Nurses know that what patients feel is possible from their perspective while they are lying in bed, is altogether different when they try to stand up and walk. In this way, somology is used by nurses to integrate lived body experience (wants) with physical possibilities (limitations of the object body), and to protect patients from themselves as it were.

Expectations about the particular trajectory for particular patients are based almost exclusively on the patient's medical condition. If, for example, the patient has a cardiac condition, or had a particular surgical procedure, the patient will be expected to follow a trajectory typical of that condition. There are routine recovery patterns for different types of conditions and surgical procedures. The management of recovery, like so many other clinical functions of nurses, however, is influenced by experience, and while it is possible to identify the salient features of the trajectory, it is much more difficult to make generalisations about how nurses manage situations when the normal trajectory is not followed. The following account from an expert nurse (in Benner's [1984] terms) illustrates that well.

I.   *I think you have a . . . norm and that's usually gauged by what you've seen over the years and if somebody doesn't fit into that you look at other things that might be wrong. It might be themselves, some people are just groaners and moaners and never want to get up and [they] have very low pain thresholds and they can't move and they are gonna take a bit longer. Then there might be other problems, like they might have secondary infections and things like that. You've got to look at all those things. That's something that you've learnt over the years.*

R.   *How does that norm become known to the patient?*

I.   *I suppose it's what we tell them. Like 'you can get up and have a shower now'. . . .*

R.   *What happens if the nurse's expectations and the patient's [expectations] are different?*

I.   *Have a confrontation, don't you. 'I don't want to get out because I'm too sore', you know. Well then I think if it's because of the fact they've been cut open – I mean, everybody's sore – anything you do. Then I think you've got to be stronger and they have to do what you say. But you've got to be very conscious how you get around it.*

R.   *But the nurse maintains control of the actions of the patient?*

I.   *I think so, yes. But then . . . experience tells you when it isn't just because they're sore and the incision. If it's something that's persistent you're looking at whether or not they've got any fistulas or abscesses, or you look at other things. And those things you usually pick up before it shows.*

General and specific trajectories in recovery

While there is one notion about the patient's generalised recovery trajectory, there are also multiple smaller trajectories which concern such things as mobility, toileting and personal hygiene. Each specific trajectory corresponds with the progressive 'handing back' of body functions, and control of them, to the patient as the patient moves toward recovery. Such shifts in control are 'recovery markers' which signify a redefinition of the level of dependence the patient has on the nurse. This is similar to shifts in control to the nurse when the patient is dying, but it is more direct (and sometimes directive) in the case of the recovering patient.

Episodes of shifting control may be acknowledged in a celebratory manner by both patient and nurse. These celebrations often concern physical events that would ordinarily be unremarkable, for example, urination or expelling flatus after surgery.

*I think we tend to brainwash patients to a certain extent [asking them post-operatively] . . . 'have you peed yet?', and until that happens you think 'we might need a catheter here'. You know, **patients have got to pee** and you don't leave them alone unless they do (laughter) and I think patients tend to get on the wavelength with you too. I mean once you get over that milestone . . . and producing the goods, quite often they can't anyway. The poor buggers are so intent in doing it that they can't . . . but it doesn't take them long to realise 'well, this is what's expected of me' and 'when I've done it, that's great'. You get past that and of course they've got to start passing wind and that's the biggest thing out and . . . you seem to need to celebrate when that happens.*

Recovery is essentially about becoming independent and regaining control over one's body functions and body care. While nurses maintain control over what the patient is expected to do during recovery, the patient progressively resumes responsibility for different body functions and aspects of body care, and nurses relinquish control over what they previously had to do **for** the patient. The significance of the compliance and control rule and the protection rule thus declines. When patients are dying, however, the markers represent decline as the patient relinquishes responsibility for body care and body functions to the nurse and 'hands over' the body.

Dying and control of the body

What control the dying patient has over daily body care does not necessarily alter the course of the dying trajectory, but it may alter the way in which the patient spends the last days or weeks of life. Nurses expect dying patients to become progressively more dependent and to require increasing amounts of assistance as they get closer to death and as they progressively 'hand over', and nurses 'take over', the body – one function at a time. This expected pattern takes place, however, in negotiation with the nurse who will usually encourage the patient to continue without assistance for as long as they possibly can.

If it's terminal [the patient's condition] I tend to let them do what they want to. If they don't feel like getting up today, well, they can stay in bed. It's not going to change anything if they stay in bed for the day or they don't want to have a shower, they can have a wash in bed or whatever.

******

It is different, because you realise . . . its a reversal [to the recovering patient], you're going to be doing more and more for them instead of less and less. I let them do what they can for as long as they can, because that's their dignity. Let them keep it. And you just expect in time you'll be doing more and more.

When a patient is dying, the rate of decline is monitored closely by nurses, family members and others who are close to the patient. The trajectory that Glaser and Strauss (1968) described was confirmed many times during the interviews I recorded. Nurses and patients' significant others have certain expectations about how long dying takes for particular patients, and those expectations structure the ways nurses define the situation. When patients take 'too long' to die the situation becomes problematic, and it can be difficult to manage, more so than is the case of the patient who dies rapidly. Often the dying patient who lingers too long is difficult to look after because the body deteriorates badly and care is difficult to maintain. There is a sense of frustration felt by nurses and relatives when a patient deviates from the dying trajectory.

*[X] was a classic case in point [and he lingered] for five days before he actually did die. . . . You get to a point where you believe with a little careful use of morph[ia] it's often not 24 hours then [before they die]. Now if, for argument's sake, it goes on for 3 or 4 days you almost become angry with the person because they didn't die when they should have. . . . You see that **so much.** It's quite one of the hardest things.*

******

If they [dying patients] go on for too long they [the nurses] get pissed off . . . because they think he should have gone last week, he's a bloody nuisance now . . . and the family start to say 'he's Dad, and I love him, but it would be a blessing if he died tonight' . . . or they come and ask [us] all the time . . . to put a specific time of death on the person because they want it to end too.

Just as it is not 'normal' for patients to linger too long, it is also not expected that they should give up, 'hand over' the body, and dislocate themselves from the usual pattern of life during their dying. Patients are expected to retain a level of control over their dying. During the course of my interviews an incident occurred in one hospital which greatly impressed and shocked the nurses, because of the amount of control they saw one woman assume over her dying. Her story is worth telling because it is an extreme illustration of how nurses respect the control patients are encouraged to have over their bodies as they die. The woman had gone to hospital to die and did not expect to take too long doing it, nor to lose control in the process. On admission she looked a little pale, but otherwise healthy, affluent and attractive. She died within three days, apparently because that was what she wanted to do.

Oh she had good control of what she wanted! ... She had her mind made up as to what she wanted. It was just good ... just to hear her rejecting things that she didn't want – and when the morphia was [suggested] – yes, she'd have that. It was clear, you could see the distinct difference [between what she would have done and would not have done]. ... That's how she wanted to go. She wanted to be still looking nice, without losing all that weight. ... She knew exactly what was going on. ... We didn't do a lot for her, and ... that's what she wanted to do. ... Fascinating.

One thing that was remarkable about this woman, in addition to her extraordinary control, was the way in which there was little evidence of physical decline. Glaser and Strauss (1968:6–7) claim nurses use physical indicators as pointers to the patient's location on the dying trajectory. The body is the signifier of dying, yet in this woman's case there was little to indicate she would soon die. One interviewee gave a graphic description of how she saw it.

I think [the people I find difficult] are the people who go on longest and suffer and their bodies show it. They actually rot. They do. They rot, but I think for me that's dreadful. (. . .) When they're sick or dying it's the body which is showing us. (. . .) It's very basic (. . .), when you've got a good body (. . .) you're dealing with simple things like cleanliness and making people comfortable. When somebody is incapacitated (. . .) that's where they are totally dependent on you.

DOING NOTHING

During this time when the patient is dying and is totally dependent on the nurse for all body care, one sometimes hears the term 'doing nothing' used to describe what is being done for the patient. I was interested to hear how nurses defined this term because it seemed to me a strange way of describing what I knew from experience to be a difficult time, emotionally and practically, for nurses, the patient and significant others. 'Doing nothing' is a term with multiple meanings.

Glaser and Strauss (1965:Chs 11 & 12) describe a time in dying which they call the 'nothing more to do' phase, at which point efforts to save the patient from dying cease, and emphasis shifts to a priority on comfort (which means physical care for the body). At this point, also, in Glaser and Strauss's (1965) description, there is a vagueness about what actually happens between the nurse and the patient, and, as a topic within their analysis, it seems to have been passed over and largely dismissed. This is possibly another illustration of their medico-dominant approach to health care and care of the dying in particular, because it emphasises a cure-oriented medical approach to illness which does not take account of nursing reality. However, it could also illustrate, among other things, that the work was not visible to the researchers because it was done in private, and they were denied access to that part of patient care.

Glaser and Strauss (1965) write about this phase of dying using a functionalist sociological approach which makes it appear self-evident that, once doctors have given up attempts to cure the patient, there is literally 'nothing more to do', and so doctors relinquish patient care to nurses. They do not see either this phase, or the nursing care of the patient's body during this phase, as problematic.

To nurses, 'doing nothing' is a term which defines a medical reality, because the patient cannot be cured by medical means, and no heroic measures will be initiated to prolong the patient's life or to prevent death from occurring (the two are not the same).

I would see that [term] in a medical sense, no resuscitation measures. Keeping them comfortable and pain free. . . . And we use the term, 'general nursing care', and definitely the term, 'doing nothing', is not the term for that.

******

It means nothing active. Nothing aimed at cure and probably nothing aimed at trying to prolong their life. . . . It's a crazy way of putting it, . . . it's not pertaining to what you're doing for that person's body.

******

Well, for me, if I hear someone say that ['doing nothing'] then obviously that patient is at the stage where there really isn't anything, medically, more that can be done and let the patient die in dignity.

The body care involved in looking after terminal patients is time consuming and difficult, and, while many nurses recognise it as one of the most demanding types of nursing, it too, like so much of nurses' work and women's work, remains largely hidden away from public view. The term, 'doing nothing', symbolises how that kind of work, which is essentially dirty work, also relies heavily on emotional labour (see Hochschild 1983), and how it is rendered invisible. If one is said to be 'doing nothing' then linguistically the work does not exist. As one interviewee put it, terminal care is 'a lot of doing something'. I will return to this theme in Chapter 10, but for now it is useful to consider accounts of what the term, 'doing nothing' means to two registered nurse who have worked extensively with cancer patients, many of whom were terminal.

I personally hate it, because I think there's still stuff we [nurses] can do for them, but it is a term that's frequently used when no more curative work can be done, like whatever you give them isn't going to cure the disease, but I think it's very erroneous and very bad to say we can do nothing for them because there is a whole heap you can do and should be doing for them.

★★★★★★

I perceive it purely as a medical thing. . . . Some days they [patients] would want to ask you questions, they would want to talk to you. You would sit down for 2 or 3 or even 4 hours with somebody. That's not nothing. Even though their treatment might have been ceased, you're still doing something.

In many ways the care of patients during their dying days or weeks, often when they are no longer able to hold a meaningful conversation, is typical of women's work. Nothing is produced from this work in that the patient will not recover. It is not highly valued work, nor work which has a high public profile. It is dirty work, and it is demanding of those who do it. In many ways it amounts to little more than physically tending the body, when patients lose the ability to talk with the nurse. One nurse summarised her perceptions of 'doing nothing' in these terms.

I think . . . nursing duties are seen as menial. What a doctor prescribes is seen as important and 'doing nothing' means doing nursing duties and the doctor will no longer prescribe anything. . . . What nurses do is not seen or valued. . . . Nurses have always been in the background – the handmaiden to the doctor — and only seen to be doing what the doctor tells them what to do. . . . So if the doctor says 'do nothing' . . . then – really all the nurses are doing is nothing. They're not assisting the doctor. They are no longer handmaiden to the doctor.

The term, 'doing nothing', and Glaser and Strauss's (1965) notion of the 'nothing more to do' phase of dying convey not only the low status of this work, they also devalue it as work. It is work which has also had the added problem of being privatised and viewed with some ambivalence in that it is menial, and it concerns death – a taboo topic. In our society, death is regarded with a mixture of emotions, and at times, superstition and fear, and this is also apparent in the ways nurses manage the dead body.

THE DEAD BODY

Nurses' management of the dead body is a rich source of information about how we deal with death. Nurses see a lot of death, they handle a lot of dead bodies in their careers, and they are probably second only to undertakers as an occupational group in being regularly exposed to dead bodies. Other occupational groups, such as ambulance officers, medical practitioners and police, also see a lot of bodies, as do people who work in morgues, but nurses see the body before and after death, and in many cases they have an established relationship with the person who has died. To the researcher, nurses are ideally placed to provide some insight into how we Australians manage death and the dead body.

In general, there are few things that can be said about how we regard death, beyond seeing it as a failure of medicine to cure disease, as is evidenced in the way dying is seen as a time of 'doing nothing' or 'nothing more to do'. And death is a time of both loss and relief, particularly if the dead person has suffered. We are a society that has tended to privatise death and to regard talk of it as taboo (Feifel 1963, Faberow 1963), and it has been largely ignored as a topic for research. We are also a society which has so-called 'respect' for the dead, but this is a problematic notion.

Respect for the dead

Respect for the dead is deeply embedded in our culture, and many of the nurses I interviewed told me they treat the body 'with respect' when they prepare it for transport to the morgue, and when they handle it generally. One registered nurse illustrated what 'respect' meant when he physically handled the body.

> . . . you still have respect for that body, the way you're washing it and you're not doing it carelessly, dropping parts. You're treating it as a person. Sort of respecting their person, even though they're dead, kind of thing. You're sort of doing it in a careful way, even though they're dead. That's how I see it. I couldn't just throw it round as a corpse as though it doesn't matter any more.

To some nurses, handling the dead body is no different from handling the living body, and they treat it in the same way they would if the person was alive, handling it carefully and talking as though the person is still there. To them it is not just a body, because the body symbolises what we do not know of death. To others death presents emotional difficulty if not a sense of disturbance.

I just feel I cut out emotionally. A dead body – you wash them and clean them before they go to the morgue. I feel very uncomfortable. I don't like the experience, whereas I don't have that problem with someone who's living. . . . I think it's just the fact that they're dead. They've been lost. That again depends on why they're dead too. I mean, I've laid out bodies where I've been glad they're dead, but it still leaves an emptiness when I'm washing them. And I guess just the unknown – the unknown aspects of death.

Others treat the dead body as a thing – an object which has ceased to have status as a person, but still they treat the body with respect.

I know a lot of people who are concerned about how you treat bodies after they die. For me, after they've died it is a body.

Nurses' perceptions of death

The crucial elements in how nurses treat the dead body seem to be based on how they themselves see death and what they believe takes place at death. The reason(s) why the death occurred is also important, as is the age and manner of death, and nurses' approach to individual deaths depends on whether or not they had an existing relationship with the person who has died. The importance of this relationship is illustrated well by those whose jobs have brought them into contact with many dead bodies, and they can compare their responses when they have or have not known the person.

I think immediately when someone dies and you have to attend to them, you have to regard them as the same person to be looked after. You don't – you couldn't – disconnect from them, that quickly. You know, your old DOAs you wouldn't know very much about them . . . We used to scrub them and lay them out. You could be doing anything – cleaning out the kitchen sink. But [for] a person you'd been nursing . . . you would feel a lot more sadness. Then again I used to feel very sorry for the old derelicts. They had no-one to mourn them. I don't think anyone deserves to die without someone to mourn them.

★★★★★★

R.   *When you're dealing with a dead body, do you regard it as a body, or Mr X?*

I.   *Depends how long I knew him.*

R.   *If you knew him well?*

I.   *It's quite difficult, because he's still sort of there, it's still him. If I hardly knew him he's a body.*

R.   *And they're easy to deal with?*

I.   *Quite easy to deal with. MVAs . . . – they were brought in off the street and they would raise very little emotion.*

R.   *You had no relationship?*

I.   *No. No relationship with anyone.*

R.   So it was easy?
I.   Yes.

One of the most intriguing aspects of this research is the extent to which death and the dead body invoke a deep sense of uncertainty bordering on superstition in some nurses to the extent that some have difficulty touching dead bodies. About one third of the interviewees talked about their feelings of uncertainty about death, most of which relate to what possibly happens after death.

For my sanity I want to play it the way I want to play it. I always make sure that if I'm sponging someone who is dead then I have someone else with me. It's still quite frightening, I think. One minute life, next minute – that's it. . . . I find it fairly distressing. . . . After each one I tend to switch off a bit.

★★★★★★

I don't cope with death terribly well . . ., it's kind of like the great unknown.

★★★★★★

The more I investigate the numerology stuff, the psychic stuff . . . the more I become aware that the spirit hangs around the body for up to 3 days. That was incorporated in Aboriginal burial customs and we as a western society don't take any notice of any spiritual considerations at all, in fact someone might die in a nursing home and the bed's occupied in 12 hours almost. . . . I feel a bit iffy about all that.

The spiritual aspect of death seems to be particularly important for some and it is related to the unknown and as yet unknowable aspects of life after death.

I've worked in places where you leave the body for an hour after they'd died so the spirit can leave the body. . . . I don't know whether there is a life after death, or whether there's not. If I choose to believe it that's fine and if I choose not to believe it, that's fine too. I mean, no-one knows. . . . We talk about patients who are unconscious and they can hear and . . . people have reported on that. I'm waiting to see the research on what happens when somebody dies – people that have cardiac arrests say they can feel themselves out of their body; they can recall looking down seeing everybody doing it. Is that something? That person is essentially dead. They are then resuscitated. What happens when you die? No-one ever comes back and says 'I could look down and see you all too'. You just don't know. You just don't know.

When they have to deal with dead bodies nurses are aware of the expectation that they should do what has to be done with respect but often their composure deserts them and they tell of such incidents in 'dead body stories'. It seems everyone has a story to tell about their particular episode where someone started to giggle over a dead body and the situation developed into something of a farce.

Uncontrollable laughter is common in these situations as is the sense of uncertainty and fear. The laughter nurses experience at these times, however, is not the same sort of laughter that occurs in everyday life, it is a form of coping behaviour which is often unintended and spontaneous. It is a nervous sort of laughter often initiated by the sometimes mechanically difficult task of handling the dead body or by unexpected happenings. For example, dead bodies often groan when they are moved and this can be sufficient to set off spasms of laughter. Although they feel as though they should not laugh because it is inconsistent with showing 'respect' it releases tension and helps them manage their discomfort.

I know that people have told stories about dropping dead people off trolleys onto the floor and laughed and joked and tried to get them into a plastic bag and this sort of carry on. I have, in that situation, laughed a couple of times, but I do think that it [laying out the body] is the last thing I will do for that person, particularly if I've nursed them for a long time. I think I would hate someone to roll me around like a sack of potatoes once I'd died. . . . The only time I have ever been what I would call inappropriate and laughed in that situation . . . was at [X] children's hospital and I think if I hadn't laughed and joked I'd have been a wreck. And I think that's how I dealt with that. And too many times in that sort of situation if you were serious and didn't laugh, didn't joke, then you would spend a lot of you time crying.

✶✶✶✶✶✶

I think as I've got older I've probably learned to have more respect for the dead. When you're 18, 19, 20 you think you're immortal anyway, that it's never going to be you there and even if it was a young person that you were laying out you tended to joke the situation away. You used a cynical form of humour so you tended to use that to get yourself through the situation anyway.

These accounts illustrate that even for those who deal with death regularly it is especially problematic if the dead body is young. There is a felt need to 'show respect', which effectively means that one deals with the situation with dignity and seriousness, this is not a time for laughter and joking, although such behaviour is necessary to avoid other responses which might be more socially disabling, in respect of getting done what needs to be done. But in laughing, there is a sense of not behaving appropriately. Death is not perceived as a time for laughter; it is a time to be serious; it is also a time surrounded by great discomfort about what it really means to be dead. Is there a life hereafter? Do patients know what you do to them after death? What does it feel like to be dead? Why do nurses often laugh during times when they handle dead bodies? Why should some people be afraid to touch the dead body? Why does the body suddenly become lifeless and what happens metaphysically when death occurs? Why do some nurses see the body of the dead person as just a body, and why do some still see it as the body of a particular person with whom they still feel a link? Why do nurses all appear to have **their** particular dead body stories? Why do they feel guilty if they do not show respect for the dead?

The 'dead body story' that emerged from this research which most aptly summarises the fear and guilt associated with lack of respect for the dead, and which lies at the base of nearly all the stories they tell is this one. It is a so-called 'morgue story' of which nurses have many. This one relates an incident that occurred one night after the nurse and a colleague had delivered a body to the morgue.

At [a Catholic hospital morgue] we had this big statue of Our Lord, Our Lady and . . . Jesus on the cross – all had beautiful big glass eyes you see. Anyhow we looked at them, we checked the fridges out to see who we knew and what not and all of a sudden we go to get out and we realised the wardsman had locked us in and that's the last I remember because I fainted. All you could see were all these glass eyes because the light went out, you see, and there were these eyes just glaring at us and we felt really wrong – like we shouldn't have gone through the fridges.

Death, dying, and the dead body are areas which are not often discussed in our culture, and from the accounts related here it would seem that we do not have a highly integrated symbolic system of dealing with death. There was no generalised pattern which emerged from this study that could summarise our approach to this area of social life, other than to say it is a time when it is not appropriate to be anything other than serious and dignified. One is supposed to treat the dead body with respect because our culture views death with respect and fear.

As a technologised and scientised society, where answers to many questions can be pursued through science, understanding the experience of death, as opposed to dying, is methodologically and logically beyond us. We have no way of knowing what happens after death unless we take on religious explanations. Additionally, death remains something of a taboo topic in western cultures, where there is emphasis on youth and beauty. It is not surprising, therefore, that nurses should share some of the fears and uncertainties about death.

Death and the dead body are a problem for nurses. By its lifelessness, the dead body underlines the interrelatedness of bodily form and personhood and it symbolises our mortality. The recovering patient, however, who is more subject to rules and expectation and control, symbolises something different. Nurses seem to have a binary approach to recovery and death – it is an either/or construction which governs expectations about the complex social patterns of recovery, dying, and the management of the body during these times.

Death has been privatised along with other aspects of life and living. In the process of this privatisation, death has become secreted away from public view as have other features of corporeal existence, and as a consequence of that process people who work with the dying and the dead have had their work privatised and removed from public view. Because nurses' work involves death and dying as well as privatised aspects of the living and recovering body, nurses' work is problematic. The only other aspect of social life and work which is similarly difficult for nurses is the relationship between sexuality, the body, and nursing care.

9. Sexuality, the body and nursing

This chapter outlines how nurses maintain the fragile context of nursing practice when they perform body care for others – acts which break many normal social rules about touch, body exposure, sexuality and sexual behaviour. The discussions build on the previous chapters by specifically illustrating how nurses deal with situations which could potentially have sexual meaning, why male sexuality is a particular issue for nursing practice, the ways in which nurses manage when patients define a situation sexually, and sexual harassment by patients.

The relationship between sexuality and the body is a central consideration of everyday practice for nurses for two interrelated reasons, both of which are derived from our constructions of sexuality and sexualised embodiment (as Chapter 4 outlined). First, male sexuality and masculinity are genital and physical constructs to a greater extent than is the case for female sexuality and femininity. Second, the genitalia are not normally exposed or touched in social life except in sexual encounters, but nurses are required to touch and handle these areas of the body as part of their work. Furthermore, we live and work in a patriarchal society in which some types of work, such as nursing, are constructed on notions of 'normal' female roles and femaleness. Because of these reasons there are difficulties experienced by nurses where male patients are concerned in this aspect of their work.

Skill is required by the nurse to construct a context in which it is permissible to see other people's nakedness and genitalia, to undress others, and to handle other people's bodies. The difficulties lie in the sensitive construction of a context in which such actions are performed, in managing situations to exclude or minimise the possibility that the patient may define the context sexually, and in managing situations where such sexual definitions are made by patients.

SEXUALITY AND THE CONTEXT OF NURSING

It is often a very delicate matter to attend to patients' needs for comfort and physical care in such a way that it is not sexually defined. As one interviewee said, patients have 'got to realise some needs cannot be met by the nurse!' Nurses take purposeful measures to manage such situations. Firstly, there is the expectation by nurses that what they do as nursing care ought not be defined by patients as a sexual experience.

*I found it most difficult to cope with . . . the men who drew sexual inferences as you did what you had to do. That made it **very** difficult. If you had somebody who played the game and went along with you it made it a lot easier. If you had someone who laid back there and leered at you and made comments about how enjoyable it was, that made it **much** more difficult.*

Secondly, much nursing care is sensual in nature, it is designed for physical comfort, and it necessarily involves touching the bodies of others in soothing and relaxing ways. Sensuality, however, is an aspect of human experience which is continuous with, and part of, many other experiences including sexual arousal, relaxation, comfort, and trust – and relaxation, comfort and trust are component parts of an ambiance of mutual sexual expression.

Patients sometimes become sexually aroused as a result of nursing care procedures and with male patients this is patently signified by an erect penis. While female patients may have similar sensual and sexual experiences during nursing care, it is not as obvious as it is with males. Patients can be embarrassed and confused as a result of that arousal for various reasons. They may not have had the experience of being cared for physically during adult life, the context is inappropriate for a sexual encounter, and, as the literature suggests, they have most likely not had many areas of the body touched outside a sexual context (see Chapter 4). This (lack of) experience can affect situations in which the patient receives care from a nurse.

It's so foreign to what most people ever dream. . . . The only contact you have physically is either sexual or you do it yourself. There is no in-between is there? People get very awkward.

Thirdly, nurses deliberately construct context by 'the manner' (see Chapter 6) and other contextors when they approach the patient for a procedure which involves sexualised parts of the body.

I.   *Well that can depend on your attitude also, and how **you** handle them, and 'handle' them also (Laughter).*

R.   *Can you give me an example?*

I.   *Well if you're washing a young virile male you're certainly not going to*

give him the come-on while you're washing his penis are you?
(Laughter) Then he might read things into it that aren't there at all.

R.   *So there is a way for nurses to go about their business that is quite*
     distinctly business.

I.   *Yes!*

Context construction in potentially sexual situations is crucial and methods which nurses employ generally are especially important when sexually invasive procedures are concerned. The following account describes how that is done.

I think it's managed by a very matter-of-fact approach. For example, coming into the room and . . . turning on the fluorescent lights making it a very clinical atmosphere, and the matter-of-fact approach, doing things with . . . two people [nurses present]. . . . Rather than if I was in bed and someone was rubbing my back it would hopefully be with a glass of champagne and dim lights. You know, it's the atmosphere, and . . . if you watch the way that nurses rub backs, . . . there would be a lot for whom it would not be a sexual act. Some [nurses] can be fairly rough.

Nursing care as a sexual experience

For some nurses, the potential for nursing care to be sensual and sexually arousing is perceived as a continuum which depends on how ill the patient is. There is a point in the patient's illness when sensuality and sexuality are not issues to be considered because the patient is too ill for those things to be relevant. It is like embarrassment – if the patient is very ill, experiences of a sexual or embarrassing nature are overtaken by the seriousness of the patient's condition. However, patient responses to nursing care which are potentially embarrassing or sexually sensitive can indicate location on a recovery trajectory and in that sense a sexual response can be a recovery marker.

I.   *Sometimes there is a difference . . . in how ill the person is, whether it*
     [nursing care of the body] is pleasurable or something that has to be
     done. It might make them feel better, but they gain no sexual
     gratification. . . .

R.   *But there's a continuous line between the sensual and the sexual?*

I.   *Yes, and to my way of thinking they move between it according to how*
     ill they are, and certainly as they recover it moves more toward the
     sexual. . . . Look, for example, at the person who is in hospital with a
     fractured femur. They are not really ill, they are just inconvenienced.
     That sort of situation is very heavily . . . toward the end of the
     continuum of sensual-sexual, but the person who comes in with multiple
     trauma . . . is beyond sex. . . . There's a line and as they move through
     from the illness through to the wellness type thing that moves them . . .
     through the sensual-sexual type thing.

There appears to be a high level of tolerance and acceptance among nurses that much of what they do as nursing care of the body is a sensual experience and that it therefore has the potential to be sexually arousing for the patient. Some nurses expect to see such responses in some types of patients, especially those who have been seriously ill or hospitalised for a long time. Orthopaedic patients, for example, were singled out by most of the nurses I interviewed as patients for whom sexuality is particularly problematic. However, situations where the patient defines nursing care of the body as **primarily** sexual threatens the nurse's construction of nursing practice.

Just to make them [patients] a bit more comfortable, even though some are up and around, you give them a back rub. But some men get to the point – they're up and about, they're showering, they don't really need back rubs but they'll ask you for a back rub and I think then it's only because of their little ego trip, or thrill they're getting out of it. . . . After a while I don't offer it.

Nurses accept that sexuality is part of human life and they expect some sexual expression on the patient's part, although within taken-for-granted social norms and the contexts of hospitalisation and nursing care. Sometimes nurses create opportunities for patients to have a sexual experience while in hospital, although such situations are uncommon and when they do occur they are usually not publicised.

I remember the night [X] let the woman into bed with her husband and Dr. [Y] came in the next day and . . . went crook. . . . He said 'you know sex is the most exhausting thing and I told you to keep him quiet'. And [X] said 'I was looking after other parts!. This fellow's in plaster'.

The major difficulty, for the (female) nurse, in dealing with the potentially sexual aspects of nursing care, arises in situations where she is the object of sexual expression, and which she may (or may not) call sexual harassment, for example, where the patient's behaviour breaks the taken-for-granted rules, particularly the modesty rule. This is most likely to occur at times when nursing care involves the genitalia, in particular the male genitalia. There is an assumed rule among nurses that 'good' patients do not embarrass the nurse by deliberately behaving sexually during nursing care.

THE MALE GENITALIA AND NURSING

As Chapter 4 outlined, the body's genital regions are heavily invested with meaning about the nature of sexuality and gender and the male body, particularly the penis, is especially invested with symbolism about the power of men. The penis is the central anatomical feature which illustrates male power and consequently nursing acts involving the penis require careful social management. Further, the sexualised construction of the body and our cultural prohibitions on touching the genitals of another person present the nurse with several socially delicate areas of practice.

Obviously the big toe is not as difficult as dealing with someone's bowel, or vagina, or penis, or whatever.

The work of Jourard (1966, 1967), and Jourard and Rubin (1968) (discussed in Chapter 4) illustrates that the genital areas of the body are virtually taboo to touch in social life. Where nursing practice is concerned, however, such taboos must be broken, and this is one of the earliest things nurses learn through experience. Despite that experience, the male genitalia continue to be problematic, and nurses do not easily overcome a primary socialisation which proscribes touching other people's genitals. While nurses may become more comfortable about their own feelings, they constantly encounter people who are hospitalised for the first time and require nursing assistance with body care. We live in a clothed society and that means we are not accustomed to seeing or touching other people's genitals or genital regions, nor allowing them to be seen or touched by other people.

You wear clothes because you get arrested if you don't.

******

We don't often expose ourselves in full nudity, we have doors on our toilets, we even get embarrassed sometimes at advertising for toilet tissues and any sanitary or hygienic products that we use or maintain our personal hygiene. . . . In my limited exposure to sexual intimacy with another human being I've found that . . . people are not inclined to get their gear off.

Nurses' access to the unclothed body of the patient is usually only a socially awkward problem when it necessitates exposing and/or handling the genitalia, or when the patient is exceedingly modest.

Touching the penis

Situations when nurses must handle genitalia, especially the penis, must be carefully managed because embarrassment can be acute and the social environment can become very awkward and fragile. Handling such areas of the body can be especially embarrassing when nurses are inexperienced and still learning to overcome their primary socialisation which incorporates notions about the private nature of the body and some body functions. The account below outlines how one nurse was given advice by her colleagues (in the 1960s) about how to socially manage catheterising a man.

I was told 'for God's sake, whatever you do, don't touch it, make sure you use a sterile towel or something and don't dare touch it' . . . because that was just too embarrassing for both you and the person and it might cause an erection. . . . And the other piece of advice from a fairly humorous person was that she dealt with it by piling a stack of pillows on the man's abdomen so . . . you couldn't actually see each other's faces.

This advice is similar in many respects to much of what I heard during my interviews. Nurses will use a number of techniques, for example, wearing gloves, to avoid touching the penis, particularly with their bare hands, and they also use social methods to help them manage. It is a persistently awkward area of nursing and one which is the subject of much informal education and discussion among nurses. One nurse, who is now very experienced, described how she and her colleagues washed male bodies and the genitalia, in particular, when they first started their careers.

I.   *You never washed it [the genitalia]. You washed down as far as it and you came up as far as it, and then you gave them the soapy washer if they were able to and then you always had to go and get something.*
R.   *And what if people weren't able to wash it?*
I.   *You washed it – as quickly as you could! And talked! While you did it – about anything that came into you head. (Laughter)*

With experience, however, nurses become less embarrassed by having to handle male genitalia, although they recognise that the patient may be very embarrassed in requiring such assistance, and they become less impressed by the apparent power of masculinity vested in the penis. Acute embarrassment on the part of the patient, however, is a problem for the nurse, and it seems that men in their 60s and older can be especially prone to very acute embarrassment.

I had a dear old bloke not very long ago and I don't believe in exposing people any more than necessary and I've always been one to cover them up, but this fellow wanted his handkerchief, he's grabbing for his handkerchief, and I said to him, 'what do you want your handkerchief for?', and he said 'I've got to cover it'. I said 'cover what?', and he said 'cover it'. And this fellow was in his late 60s and I said 'I'm not going to expose you unnecessarily, I will keep you covered', but he had to have that handkerchief. . . . We were doing battle over the handkerchief but he kept his hand there all the time, and I don't know whether he'd had a nasty experience at some stage or not – (laughter) – and here I am a mature woman – very, very difficult it

*was because I don't know whether he had a proper wash the whole time he
was there.*

★★★★★★

I.   *Old farmers who've always done for themselves . . . are highly
     embarrassed and say 'you shouldn't have to do this sort of thing for me',
     or [they are] protective or unwilling to have the sheet removed . . . and
     they do not like young girls, and that could be anyone from me [in my
     40s] to a young girl, having to do for them.*
R.   *But it's alright to clean their teeth?*
I.   *Yes!*

Accidental erections

One of the major difficulties in dealing with male genitalia is the
possibility that the penis will become erect as it sometimes does
during nursing care. Such situations require particularly sensitive
social management on the nurse's part in order to continue to
define the situation as a nursing event and not a sexual event. If the
patient is perceived to be embarrassed and the erection is perceived
as 'accidental', the nurse will interpret the situation as one in which
the patient did not intend 'anything to happen'. There is, therefore,
no intentional rule-breaking. However, if the patient appears to be
interpreting the situation as a sexual encounter, or to be enjoying
the event, the nurse may feel professionally compromised and/or
harassed and respond accordingly.

Unintended erections are usually managed sympathetically and
sensitively by the nurse using a variety of strategies. These include
taking time out, using their learned lack of affect to define the
situation as manageable and unremarkable, or ignoring the fact
that the patient is having an erection.

*Occasionally . . . a man has had an erection. . . . That isn't pleasant for us
and he's embarrassed too. . . . Put a towel over it and come back later. . . .
Sometimes discretion is probably better than making an issue of it.*

★★★★★★

I just pretend it's not there. I just pretend it's not happening.

★★★★★★

*I did have an embarrassing situation one day taking out stitches. He'd had
varicose veins [removed] and I got half way up the groin and he got an
erection. I said 'oh, I think someone's calling me', and I left and walked out,
did something else. When I came back he was alright. . . . I walked away
and when I came back it was all normal.*

Nurses who are male also find it necessary to manage situations when a patient has an erection during body care. This situation can be embarrassing and disturbing for the patient and the nurse. The following account illustrates how one registered nurse, who identifies himself as homosexual, manages such situations.

I.   *I've never commented, that's one thing. I have never laughed, and sometimes I could have laughed. What I've done is go on as though it [the erection] wasn't there.*

R.   *What have you been doing at the time?*

I.   *Usually washing there. And by the time the erection is at full mast I've nearly finished and you can roll them over and do [wash] their backs. . . . I mean it must be fairly embarrassing. . . . The only time it's ever happened to me was with a gay patient. I've never had it happen with a patient who was presumably heterosexual, but mostly with quite overt, open, gay men.*

The other three men in this study did not identify sexual behaviour (of male or female patients) as problematic for them, except in situations where the patient was exposing himself or herself deliberately. Like their female colleagues, male nurses do not tolerate such exposure. It is outside the boundaries of socially acceptable body exposure in public. Sexual arousal, however, of the kind outlined above, which is presumed by the nurse to be unintended, and which embarrasses the patient, is managed as a relatively routine part of nurse's work in stark contrast to sexual behaviour which is perceived to be deliberately directed at the nurse.

OVERT SEXUAL BEHAVIOUR, BODY EXPOSURE AND HARASSMENT

Overt sexual behaviour by patients (directed toward nurses) is not tolerated among nurses unless the patient has impaired judgement from illness or injury. For example, patients who suffer brain damage are usually treated with tolerance and understanding, but unnecessary body exposure, particularly exposure of the genitalia, including female breasts, and sexually suggestive talk are violations of the modesty rule at least. They can also violate another rule that nurses take for granted, that is, that the patient should not exploit nursing situations or nursing care, and may well be seen by the nurse as a form of sexual harassment. The data reported here illustrate how nurses deal with rule breaking situations in which the patient is sexually explicit.

Sexual actions directed toward female nurses almost invariably involve male patients, although two incidents were related in this study where female patients made sexually explicit advances to some male nurses, but one of those incidents involved a patient who was psychiatrically disturbed at the time, and the other was a post-partum woman (which is often an emotionally labile time). Another incident involving male harassment of a male nurse is also reported, but it concerned verbal abuse rather than a sexual advance. Advances where the female approaches the male generally take the form where the female makes known her willingness to participate in sexual activity. It is an indication of availability rather than an overt invitation or request, which characterises male advances to female nurses, and in that sense these incidents are in keeping with notions that females are passive and receptive (rather than proactive) sexually. Situations in which patients make advances to nurses would also seem to be exclusively heterosexual and to some nurses it is perceived as a form of sexual harassment.

Situations in which patients expose their genitalia to nurses in sexually suggestive ways reflect a belief that nurses tolerate such behaviour, and/or that their work involves sexual favours for the patient. In this sense, therefore, it is not simply a reflection of social attitudes of men toward women, but also a reflection of a specific stereotype of nurses. The following account, which is very explicit and possibly an extreme example, illustrates how one patient's perception of what nurses do in their work influenced his approach to the nurse.

I.   Oh this [incident] was horrific. I was a second year nurse. A fellow came in with burns to his hands and trunk. [I was] sponging him, he was a little older than us – 21, 22, and he said 'my friend told me a nurse would help me out', and I said, 'yeah, what's your problem?' [And he said] 'you know', and I said 'do you want a bottle?'. 'No, my friend told me you'd help me out' [he said] and suddenly . . . it just suddenly clicked what he meant. I just picked up the bowl and ran out and did not want to go back in that room.

R.   In his head nurses perform the functions of prostitutes?

I.   Yes.

On a less extreme level patients are sexually suggestive toward nurses and expose themselves without being as direct as the patient in the account above.

I know with one patient . . . it [erections and sexually suggestive behaviour] used to happen quite often. And I know one day he just got to me so I threw a towel at him and walked away until things cooled down and he'd settled down, and then I came back and started showering him again. . . . He wasn't embarrassed, he started being crude.

Overt sexual behaviour directed at the nurse is a common feature of nurses' work environment and one which they manage with a variety of methods. Some nurses respond to patients' sexually explicit behaviour by using jokes and humour, and they use a form of trivialisation not unlike the *minifisms* they employ in other potentially embarrassing situations. One experienced nurse related her account of the first time a patient ever showed her his erect penis and she also describes how nurses will trivialise male patients' attempts to make the nurse the object of their sexual advances.

He sort of lifted the bedclothes and said 'what do you think of this?'
(Laughter) My mother had been a nurse and she had told funny stories about this sort of thing and how to react, and her answer was 'I've never seen a good looking one yet', which was guaranteed to deflate the occasion. And I can remember not even remembering to try that – just sort of beating a hasty retreat (laughter) from the room and bursting into gales of laughter in the pan room with another nurse who was there. Now I think at [age] 40 plus, after 23 years [of nursing] sometimes it can be a little flattering in its own funny way (laughter) that they even think you're worth the effort (laughter). But the people who respond now are getting older (laughter). It's not the young ones any more. We had a funny instant the other week. A young fellow asked one of the nurses, who is the same age group as me, where the young pretty sexy nurses were this particular evening. She said 'I'll go and get one for you', and came and got me (laughter) and I told him he was much better off with an experienced person (laughter). He didn't catch the joke, but the man in the next bed, who was about 52–53, thought it was a scream (laughter).

Other methods to manage situations where patients break the rules with explicit sexual behaviour, include making their intolerance known to the patient, trivialising what the patient does, and indicating to the patient that nurses' work does not include sexual favours. Generally, but not always, such incidents are dealt with by nurses in a way that defines them as relatively harmless sexual advances rather than as sexual harassment, and a direct approach to the patient is usually used.

If the behaviour is persistent the patient's reputation is spread rapidly among the staff, who then employ mechanisms to protect each other. For example, nurses will not tend to the patient alone, and they will spend the minimum amount of time necessary to do nursing care, and, if there is a male colleague on the staff, they may ask him to help with any body care that is required for that patient. Irrespective of the methods used, the aim in these circumstances is to provide only the care which is essential. Nurses will maintain a vigilant and distant approach to the patient, particularly if his behaviour is persistent and perceived by the nurse to be sexual harassment. As well as being protective of nurses, these strategies are also designed for avoidance, and to minimise opportunities for the patient to exploit the nurse sexually. If the patient continues to be sexually explicit, the situation can be very difficult to manage, and often it is relieved only when the patient is discharged.

However, the point at which this sort of behaviour is perceived as harassment, if it is perceived that way at all by nurses, is difficult to establish. Persistent sexual approaches from the patient are difficult to manage in nursing because of the need for someone to continue to have a professional nursing responsibility for the care provided. It seems as though sexually explicit verbal advances from patients are more easily managed than physical harassment, for example, touch and stroking the nurses' leg, when she turns a patient over in bed.

When is overt sexual behaviour harassment?

The term 'sexual harassment' did not come into common usage until the 1970s and since that time we have become more aware of it as a phenomenon to be named and understood. Much of what has been reported in this chapter can alternatively be viewed as sexual harassment – it is a way of looking as a situation, a way of defining what is happening. Much of what happens to nurses in their daily work can be constructed as sexual harassment, if the person doing the perceiving choses to see things in that way. If we are to name aspects of nursing care as sexual harassment, we will subject much of nurses' work to analyses through a sexual lens – a process which may make people (including nurses) uncomfortable. Not surprisingly, therefore, sexual harassment of nurses has not been widely studied and there is only a small amount of literature on the subject. Much of that literature deals only with harassment by other staff members, particularly medical practitioners and supervisors. Very little attention has been paid to sexual harassment of nurses by patients, and what there is of that literature is problematic, as I will explain below.

The data reported in this study directly address the question of sexual harassment of nurses by patients. However, this is not an easy topic to research, for many reasons, and I collected only a small amount of data in which nurses actually used the term 'sexual harassment' to describe incidents, though much of what they reported could be termed as such. Nurses, like most women, have not readily discussed or named or made sexual exploitation explicit. In nursing there are some salient points which may indicate why this is so, and one of them is that overt sexual behaviour by patients towards nurses has been incorporated into their working lives to point where it is institutionalised as part of the job.

Nurses do not see sexual harassment as a major problem. Rather, it is perceived as an aspect of their work which they must manage from time to time, and many have become accustomed to it — and that raises other issues. As an occupational group, nurses have always encountered a level of overt sexual attention from patients and from the public. Nursing has not only been a highly sex-typed occupation, but also a highly sexualised one. The difficulty for the researcher in matters of this kind seems to lie in nurses having seen the sexualised nature of their work as part of the job, taken it for granted, and never having explicitly identified it as a topic for research, debate or discussion. It has not been problematised within the context of an occupation particularly prone to sexual exploitation, at least not in so far as patients are concerned.

It is also possible that sexual harassment of nurses by patients is a taboo topic among some nurses, and that they, therefore, do not want it researched. Jordheim (1986:32) has suggested that this could be a possible reason for the small literature on the subject, and that gatekeeping may reflect a vested interest in keeping it hidden, for fear it may tarnish the image of nurses. Despite such attempts to protect the image of nursing, nurses continue to encounter men who see them only as women (and not as professionals providing care) and behave toward them accordingly. Such men stereotype nurses as members of a particular occupational group that is highly tolerant of overt sexual behaviour or even invites and welcomes it.

I think that people think that we're used to that sort of thing. My boyfriend thinks I am. He says 'you're used to that sort of thing by now'. I think that's the general public . . . image of the nurse . . . – that because we're so used to it . . . seeing the naked body and accept it, [we] think nothing of it, whereas the general public doesn't and if they see a naked body they take a double look.

Sexual harassment and nursing ideology

One of the most important studies of sexual harassment (Collins & Blodgett 1981) illustrates that sexual harassment is essentially about the power which men use against women, although sexual harassment, is not exclusively a male-to-female phenomenon. Faley (1982) also argues that gender is fundamental in sexual harassment as is the power relationship between men and women. Both of these studies concern sexual harassment in the workplace and they direct attention to sexual harassment which women experience from fellow workers. In my study, I was interested in the issue of sexual harassment as it concerned nurses' work with body care for patients.

Where nursing practice is concerned, nurses do not necessarily identify overt sexual advances from patients as sexual harassment, although the actions in question are essentially the same as those which Collins and Blodgett (1981) identified in the workplace among fellow workers. Nurses have preferred to call such actions things other than sexual harassment, for example, 'seductive behaviour' (Assey & Herbert 1983), they have located them in the context of the care the nurse **should** give the patient, and they have discussed the issue in moralistic tones. Literature such as the Assey and Herbert (1983) paper tends to convey the impression that this is a relatively trivial matter, or one that does not really exist.

There are, however, several papers (most of them North American) which address the issue of sexual harassment as an administrative matter affecting productivity and the work environment, among other things (Duldt 1982, Elliott & Kaiser 1982, Mendelson 1983, Colantonio 1984, Murphy 1986, Creighton 1987a, 1987b) and they have ignored the issue of patients sexually harassing nurses. Creighton (1987b:16) says, for example, that 'typically in nursing, the harasser is a physician or supervisor in a position of power or superior social position, while the typical harassee is a relatively powerless staff nurse, team leader or head nurse'.

Such authors have been blind to the problems which nurses encounter from patients although there is some literature (of the recipe type) giving advice on how to manage sexually harassing patients. These papers at least make the issue explicit as a legitimate topic for debate (Hacker 1984, Arbeiter 1986, Anonymous 1986) but little empirical work has been done in this area, although sexual harassment from work colleagues and patients has been recognised in Australian nursing as an industrial issue (Ridgeway 1984a, 1984b).

It is possible that sexual harassment has been kept hidden, not only because it may tarnish nurses' image, but also because nursing ideology closely resembles Christian doctrine in many ways. Nursing has many of it roots in religious orders, and many of its professional ideals reflect that history. The ideal that a nurse should not make critical remarks about any patient, and the strong emphasis on nurses' responsibility to care, have been accompanied by an ideological stance that locates the patient beyond criticism and places a heavy burden on the nurse to tolerate harassment. A study such as mine, therefore, helps to remove the silence surrounding this issue and makes it a problem to be named and discussed, especially when the research topic concerns the intimate nature of the work which nurses do. Sexual harassment, or a sexual encounter of any kind, is an action designed for intimacy and my work is very much about intimacy among people, how that intimacy is managed and made possible, and how it is integrated into our social system.

Nurses have not systematically challenged the professional (religious) notion that one must be able to care, irrespective of the patient, the patients' behaviour, or the circumstances. To challenge the care ethic would be heretical, yet this ethic contributes to a practice environment in which sexual harassment is not openly and officially discussed, although everyone knows it occurs. There is a moral quality to this ideology which suppresses formal talk about the sexually harassing patient. It is not considered appropriate for nurses to make derogatory remarks about patients – at least officially. As an area of discourse in nursing, and one so closely related to the body and the intimacy which surrounds body care, sexual harassment and the sexual aspects of nursing have been absent or highly censored.

Assey and Herbert (1983) provide a good illustration of this pervasive ideological stance. They define 'seductive behaviour' (read sexual harassment) as behaviour which 'the nurse *perceives* as an intention to attract her, usually for the purpose of sexual activity' (Assey & Herbert 1983:531). They further claim that this sort of behaviour on the part of patients may only indicate 'a need to receive friendliness or warmth from their caregivers' or that they feel 'isolated and lonely' and may touch the nurse only for the purpose of establishing a relationship (1983:531). They also assert that the nurse should strive to understand such patients in order to better meet their needs, and the nurse is urged to see seductive behaviour as a normal response to hospitalisation (Assey & Herbert 1983). These authors also admit, however, that seductive behaviour is one method that patients use to 'demonstrate anger toward a nurse who is considered aloof or condescending' (Assey & Herbert 1983:531). The clear message in this stance is that the nurse should tolerate this behaviour because the nurse's primary role is to satisfy the needs of patients, and there is a moral imperative that she (not he) should be a 'good' nurse by understanding the patients' needs. What Assey and Herbert (1983) call 'seductive behaviour' is what others have called sexual harassment, in that it is unwelcome, uninvited, gender based, and a manifestation of the power of men over women. These authors do not see 'seductive behaviour' as problematic, and neither do they see it as essentially about male power over women. Rather, their emphasis is on what the nurse should do to minimise it, and they also claim that nurses, without realising it, may invite seductive behaviour by 'sending signals the patient perceives as seductive' (1983:532). They continue:

Nurses often straighten their posture when approaching a patient. This straightening involves tightening the abdominal muscles and putting the shoulders back, which may make the breast protrude. It is also not unusual for a nurse to place her hand on her hip or cock her head to one side while talking with the patient.

Likewise, because of the intimate nature of patient care, it is common for the nurse and patient to be in a situation that has characteristics of the stage of positioning [for courtship] (Assey & Herbert 1983:532).

The Assey and Herbert position not only takes male sexuality to be unproblematic but it also draws heavily and very selectively on Scheflen's (1965) psychoanalytic analysis of quasi-courtship behaviour which implies that: (1) virtually every act in mixed sex company is capable of having some sexual interpretation; and (2) that it is possible to unconsciously engage in courtship behaviour – an argument which takes human existence to be fundamentally, but not consciously, sexual. According to Assey and Herbert's (1983) analysis, sexual harassment (or 'seductive behaviour' as they call it) is a problem for which the nurse should find a solution, and it may well be a problem of her making. They also see it as exclusively as a male-to-female heterosexual matter. This approach appears to promote the same ideas which support the myths surrounding rape – that women who are raped invite it by wearing particular clothes or walking along the street alone at night. It also leaves three important notions unquestioned – that male sexuality is relatively uncontrollable; that women can be seen as essentially carnal creatures; that the social construction of nursing roles provides ideal opportunities for patients to be sexually expressive toward their caregivers.

Other papers about sexual harassment of nurses by patients have not regarded either male sexuality or the intimate nature of nurses' work as notions worthy of question and exploration. Jordheim (1986), for example, refers to male patients' needs to express themselves sexually, and suggests that hospitalised patients may have stronger sexual feelings because they have nothing to do all day. In similar fashion to Assey and Herbert (1983), Jordheim emphasises how nurses can learn to cope with sexual harassment and suggests that with more understanding of human sexuality, nurses will find it easier to deal with sexual harassment. She admits, however, that there is a greater potential for men to misinterpret nursing actions as sexual, particularly with the recent trends toward greater emphasis on touch and therapeutic touch.

Crull and Cohen (1984) argue that sexual harassment by patients is hidden, but they offer no explanation(s) for this even though their study revealed that it existed. Heinrich (1987) argues that sexual harassment is often confused with seductive behaviour (which she does not define) and that the patient may be responding to media images which portray the nurse as a sex object. Again, however, the emphasis is placed on what the individual nurse can do to manage the situation, and the underlying concepts of male sexuality, and nurses' work with the intimate details of bodies, are left unexplored.

SEXUAL HARASSMENT OF NURSES BY PATIENTS

The nurses I interviewed for this study, tended to see sexual harassment as irritating and annoying, and disruptive to their clinical functions, but not necessarily problematic because they have effective ways of dealing with it. One of the interviewees described in these terms;

I guess it depends on your interpretation of what's prudish and what's over-reacting. . . . They're [the patients] not considering how we feel . . . – that we might be embarrassed. . . . To me that's harassment if a fellow exposes himself. They're not considering the nurse at all.

Generally, the nurses I interviewed find it intolerable that patients should touch the nurse in sexual ways, for example, touching her breasts, or leg or that they should verbally harass the nurse. Touching the nurse is seen in a different way from situations in which patients expose themselves, probably because touch is a more invasive and intimate act. They also acknowledge that much harassment remains hidden, invisible, unidentified as harassment and unofficial.

I think a lot probably goes on that goes unreported because nurses are afraid that they might be thought to be encouraging it or something. . . . Nurses do not appreciate being mauled. . . . It shouldn't be that we're expected to put up with it.

Orthopaedic patients: sexual harassment as sport

Orthopaedic patients are particularly prone to becoming sexual harassers. Young male orthopaedic patients were singled out by the majority of interviewees as particularly prone to the initiation of sexually difficult situations. They are hospitalised for long periods, though for most of that time they are not sick, they begin to feel 'at home' in the hospital environment, and they behave as 'normal' men (what ever that means), except that they are not very mobile. They are stereotypically sexual harassers of nurses.

They feel alright, they're strung up in traction and they've got to be in bed for some time. They're not actually sick . . . they're just immobile. Who knows what's going through their minds. . . . I have seen it on four separate occasions . . . where no female was excluded . . . and it just happened that the resident [medical officer] was female and . . . the physio[therapist]. Everyone copped it . . . it was just shocking. . . . We turn around and say, you know, 'look, piss off' . . . or [if he] runs the hands up the leg well [tell him] 'don't do that, that's not nice'.

******

You've got these young guys, strung up in traction for 3 or 4 months at a time. They get a bit frustrated. ... If somebody did it [sexually harassed] once, they would never do it twice to me, whereas some other people they would pick on. But that's because you tolerate it once. You wouldn't tolerate it again. But if they're a head injury they do all those peculiar things anyway, so they really don't know what they're doing, so you've got to accept that. But if he's just a young fellow with a broken leg who makes sexual connotations all the time you just tell him, you know, 'grow up' You usually do find they grow up, or they might pick on someone else.

Orthopaedic patients provide a good illustration of the extent to which male sexuality is competitive and similar to sport. Where orthopaedic patients are located together in groups (of four, for example) this is especially apparent, and sexual harassment is one manifestation of that. It may, in fact, be the only sport available to them, because they are immobilised and virtually captive in a small environment. Orthopaedic wards can resemble other male domi- nated situations where sex-as-sport forms part of the local culture, for example, hotels, building sites and cricket fields. Considerable attention is paid to the female form and to females' responses to sexual innuendo. Patients make sexually explicit and suggestive comments to each other when one patient is receiving attention from a nurse behind drawn screens.

Not all harassment, however, is directed at female nurses. One male nurse reported being the target of considerable verbal derision from male orthopaedic patients, who called him 'a poofter' and refused to receive any nursing from him. While this is not sexual harassment in the usual sense, it is, nevertheless, interpreted by this registered nurse as such. He believes that such actions not only reveal homophobia, but that they also sex-type nursing practice in a way that can be regarded as sexual harassment, especially when patients make their bias known. In this sense, therefore, harassment is the use of male (sexual) power in a patriarchal system to impose compulsory heterosexuality (see Rich 1980) and to impose sexual metaphors on work.

SEXUALITY AND NURSING PRACTICE: A SUMMARY

Sexual harassment of nurses by patients highlights many of the sensitive and intimate aspects of nursing practice and it indicates how sexuality is constructed in our culture. Nursing practice incorporates kindness, a caring approach, warmth, gentleness and friendliness to the patient – all of which can be perceived as sexual availability if not sexual invitation, and all of which are part of the traditional caring roles of women. Nurses are meant to practise in way which emphasises that patients' needs matter. However, as women, they can become the object of sexual advances from patients, and some stereotypes of nurses promote this image of nurses and the work that they do.

The data reported here should assist in opening up the debate on the sexualised nature of embodiment and the extent to which nursing must take account of the sexualised body. That patients should at some times take advantage of nurses should not be surprising, but what is an issue to be considered is the extent to which sexual harassment and the management of the sexualised body have not been explicitly addressed as topics for nursing research. If the body is as sexualised as I have argued, then it seems only sensible that nursing should take up this issue as a central one, however, the risk here is in opening up a debate which hovers uncomfortably close the margins of respectability. It is one thing to research embodiment in illness experience – it is another matter entirely to initiate a dialogue about sexual matters as they impact on nursing practice, particularly because nurses have tried to overthrow their heavily sexualised public image.

Nurses are stereotyped as sex objects, among other things, as the considerable literature on their image indicates (see, for example,

Kalisch & Kalisch 1982a, 1982b, 1985, Kalisch et al 1982). Nurses make special provisions to manage that image, their work, and the stereotypes that people have of them, because a very considerable amount of nurses' work overlaps behaviours which in other contexts would have elements of traditional female roles – mothering, housekeeping, catering, and cleaning – all of which are service oriented and which incorporate elements of social life where women serve men (and others).

In many ways, nursing practice mirrors the way(s) men relate to women in patriarchal society, and in 'civilised' society where the body and sexuality have been privatised. Sexual harassment of nurses by patients is a reflection of the sexual exploitation of women generally.

In nursing, sexual harassment is an essentially heterosexual matter. Even though there are allegedly large numbers of homosexual nurses, and I interviewed some for this study, (homo)sexual harassment in which sexual invitations or advances are made between nurses and patients of the same sex is (reportedly) extremely rare. One interviewee explained this in terms of a dominant heterosexual ideology thesis.

There are important differences in the way homosexuals and heterosexuals define sexual contexts. In heterosexual life, sexuality is a pervasive aspect of social life and almost any situation is a potential occasion for sexual expression. For the homosexual, however, there are particular and specific places when it is acceptable to be sexually expressive and active. Those places and contexts are learned within the homosexual subculture. The heterosexual, however, has a more ill-defined set of surroundings in which it is acceptable to be sexually expressive and almost any behaviour is open to a sexual interpretation. The high level of mutual recognition among homosexuals and the more proscribed contexts for sexual expression in the homosexual subculture would seem to minimise the potential for a homosexual to harass a nurse.

The difficulty for nursing, however, which differentiates it from other forms of women's work, is the extent to which nurses' work brings them into such sustained and intimate contact with bodies and the privatised aspects of social life, including sexuality. They see life 'in the raw' so to speak. Much of nurses' work is, therefore, open to misinterpretation, like so much of women's lives. The next chapter discusses how nurses manage their work and image in their social lives beyond the work environment.

10. Nurses' work, the body and society

In their daily work and lives, nurses take for granted a sociology of the body that meets the criteria which Turner (1984) argues are needed for an adequate theory of the body. Turner (1984:38–41) claims that the essential elements of such a theory are that it must be interactive and take account of body-self dialectic, it must differentiate the individual from the population, it must accommodate the interfaces between biology and culture and between the self and society, and it must be political so as to accommodate deviance and social control. Nurses do all of these things in their practice because: (1) they take account of body-self dialectic as they manage their own physiological and affective responses to the body, and by making it possible for patients to also manage; (2) the management of the body is essentially and fundamentally an interactive and interpretive process between nurse and patient and it is negotiable; (3) nurses differentiate self from the other (and the masses) by emphasising the context of **this** patient as unique in a particular context; (4) nursing is essentially and fundamentally about the interface of the biological and the social as people reconcile the lived body with the object body during illness experience; and (5) the body, as nurses know it, is a political construct with respect to both the male body and sexuality and the invisibility of their work in patriarchal and 'civilised' society. To nurses, however, the body also has time and space and it is viewed with a form of integration that Turner (1984) does not mention, but which is fundamental to an ability to deal simultaneously with biological and social aspects of being.

NURSING WORK AND CONCEPTS OF PRACTICE

I have argued here that nurses practise in a somological way, that this is a style of practice which integrates lived experience with the

215

object body, and that somology is not necessarily holistic (taking the term to mean that the whole is greater than the sum of its parts). Somology is a composite perspective developed from what is regarded by nurses as relevant. It can be holistic but need not be, it is fundamentally person related (a common-sense definition of holism), and it is context bound. It is a view developed in practice. It is a way of knowing which is different from abstract knowledge.

In recent decades, particularly since the 1970s, nursing writers have philosophised, theorised, and proselytised 'holistic practice'. Such an approach to practice is promoted in the belief that it ensures more individualised and more personalised care. It is also believed to provide an avenue through which nursing could move away from the dominant medical model. This trend emphasises the need to see 'the whole person' (what ever that means), but it is not necessarily grounded in empirical work or practice. Rather, the trend has grown out of a perceived need to enhance nursing practice, to raise its status, to make it more humanisticly oriented, and to professionalise and scientise the occupation.

It was also a very 'clean' image of nursing to promote. The body care and dirty aspects of nurses' work disappear, to be replaced by neologisms and euphemisms. Body care is subsumed into a range of nurse-identified needs of the patient. This period in nursing can be seen as an attempt to both overcome 'the problem of the body' in an occupation of dirty workers who deal with the messy details of physical being, and to scientise and sanitise nursing knowledge and practice.

There have been some other unfortunate consequences of this trend to clean up nursing, not the least of which has been the tendency for nurses to pry into an increasing number of things in patients' lives, in order to get a more 'holistic' picture of the patient. But greater surveillance (which is what some of these actions are), and more emphasis on measurement and monitoring, neither ensures holism nor a holistic view of the patient. It may lead to more information being collected without necessarily informing or improving practice.

The trend toward more holistic care and the adoption of new terminology have not been universally embraced, particularly among experienced practitioners – the sort of people I interviewed for this study. These people have remained sceptical about such things as the nursing process and nursing diagnoses – instruments believed to foster holistic and scientific practice. They regard them as imposed models that do not reflect the real world of practice as they perceive it, experience it and practice it. Such imposed models are also reductive and they fragment an otherwise integrated and composite (somological) view which typifies the practice of experienced and expert nurses.

In none of the recent trends to better document or understand nursing practice has the body been explicitly addressed, even though it is fundamental in nursing care and a more general problem in our society for those who work with the body.

In the hospital environment and within the context of hospitalisation, many contextors are available to socially construct nurses' work so that their regular violations of normal social rules are acceptable. But as members of society nurses must manage their occupational identity in social life – outside their work environments and without access to the contextors which make their work permissible.

Nurses require a common sense knowledge of the body because much of what they manage in body care is predicated on particular social (and biological) norms about the body, its exposure, and its accessibility. Because the body and its functions are also a source of embarrassment and dirt, nurses must manage their occupational status and identity in social life outside the hospital environment as well as inside it. They must manage being a nurse in a society which proscribes touching some parts of other people's bodies and talking about body dirt.

THE PRIMACY OF THE NURSE'S IDENTITY

The identity of 'nurse' is so powerful that it can structure social interactions, and some nurses find that people respond to them, not as individual persons, but as nurses. The identity of 'nurse' is complex and it has multiple meanings and stereotypes, some of them dichotomous. However, they all centre around the intimacy which nurses have with other people's bodies, sexuality, and the problematic nature of the body in western culture. Within the context of the hospital, the nurse's identity helps to provide access to peoples' bodies and define otherwise awkward situations as socially permissible, but that same identity and the images of the nurse need management by nurses in wider society.

*They don't think of you as anything **but** a nurse, you don't have any real social life other than being a nurse. . . . I suppose what I don't like is [that] someone will be sick [vomit] and they'll say 'you won't mind, you're a nurse', or someone tells a dirty joke and says 'it doesn't matter, you're a* *nurse'. Because you're a nurse and see bodily functions [they think] you're naturally someone to whom they can make rude remarks. They forget you're a person first and a nurse second.*

Nursing is not well understood.

Among those I interviewed there was widespread consensus that nursing is not a well understood occupation in society generally, that a high level of ignorance exists about the work of nurses, and that people tend to focus on the aesthetically unpleasant or sexually related aspects of nursing practice. Nurses are often perceived primarily as people who deal with dirt, so that other aspects of their practice, particularly the somological aspects, are ignored or subsumed by an emphasis on the taboos which nurses are allowed to violate. While nurses find that their lives are sometimes complicated as a result of these images and ideas, they also understand that such ignorance originates in perceptions of what they do as work.

I think people are probably fairly ignorant of . . . what nurses do. I know many a comment has been made to me by friends 'how on earth do you deal with people's bodies?' . . . When you try to say to people outside that you don't actually look upon bodies as a physical thing people find that very hard [to accept] . . . People tend to think that you centre in on all the appropriate points [of the body] when you look at everybody. . . . They find it very hard to think that you don't have any of those thoughts whatsoever, you don't even look at those [highly sexualised] bits. I think the only people who probably understand are the people who have had the experience [of being nursed] themselves . . . and they'll say 'I don't know how you do these things, you're just wonderful'.

******

I know . . . that some people think 'how can you do that?' because they feel so embarrassed even thinking about it, you know. And my neighbour often says 'I don't know how you can stand it'. To them it's revulsion. . . . It's almost as if we're being put down for doing it. . . . It's a mixture because if you only focus on that point, well, there's obviously a stigma. But if you focus on the other work that nurses do . . . things are mixed.

One nurse overcame the problem of people's ignorance about nursing and images of nurses by emphasising that she was a midwife rather than a nurse. For her it overcame the problem of being seen as one who did dirty work – a perception which she believed came from an association with the body care work that nurses do.

When you say 'I'm a midwife', it's got a bit of glamour about what it is. . . . Nurses clean up dirty messes and . . . although it's changing, it's still very much there. If people ask me what I do now, I never say 'I'm a nurse', I always say 'I'm a midwife'. And they say 'Oh' [pleasantly]. That's fine.

Identity and nurses' work

Not only does the identity of nurse have a primacy in social relations, but the work of nurses is seen to have a primacy in those aspects of body care and body products which we have privatised in 'civilised' society. We have no socially acceptable ways to talk about these functions or some parts of the body and sexuality. That lack of space for discourse is also a problem for nurses.

I think people . . . look lowly upon us because we do things that are considered just not done I guess. Nurses are looked upon as masseurs. . . . My husband just has to mention that he's married to a nurse and they think 'oh yes'. . . . We do invade the body, we do see things that another person on the street wouldn't see.

★★★★★★

I defend my job a lot. When you get into a conversation and they start talking about looking at a patient's body, 'you must see a lot', they say. Some people can be a bit crude in conversation. . . . I think they're only fishing around to find out what you do do. Unless they've been a patient in hospital and been on the receiving end they don't really know.

In effect, therefore, nurses' work is publicly and socially constructed on the basis of its lack and its invisibility. It is not highly visible work, some people prefer to remain ignorant about it, it has low status, it concerns things regarded with an element of smut, and all of this is compounded by a reluctance of nurses to talk openly about their work.

Talking about their work

Nurses find it very difficult, if not impossible, to talk about their work with anyone other than nurses, and this is a direct result of the extent to which their work involves aspects of life which are considered dirty or which are too close to aspects of sexuality for some people's comfort. In this respect, therefore, nurses conceal their work as do others who do work designated as dirty (see Chapter 1). Their work is kept from public discussion because the nature of that work is not in itself a legitimate topic of conversation. In Foucault's (1985a, Gordon 1980) terms, therefore, there is a problem of power/knowledge located in the inability to discuss the body, or what nurses' work with the body involves.

*You can't even tell your husband. I can't, you know. . . . He wouldn't understand. You might be washing a young boy and he has an erection because he's young. How do you tell your husband something like that? . . . He doesn't want to know. So how do you tell him? So you keep it inside of you. . . . We [nurses] go through a lot of things together that other people would **never** go through and never understand, so you just talk to each other which socially isolates you a bit.*

Talking to other nurses about their work is a common method which nurses use to make what they do manageable for them as individuals. They need to talk to their colleagues because few people outside the occupation can understand what it is like to be a nurse.

[Some of what nurses do is] not the sort of thing you invite people in for afternoon tea and discuss. (Laughter) I don't think you could cope with nursing if you couldn't talk to your colleagues about what's happened, and what you've done and what you've had to do.

★★★★★★

I don't talk about the dirty messes I have to clean up. I don't talk about things like . . . somebody had the biggest set of breasts you've ever seen. No. I don't talk about other people's bodies.

There are various reasons why nurses do not easily talk to non-nurses about what they do, but they all concern 'the problem of the body', its functions, and other taboo topics, such as sexuality and death. In not talking about their work nurses are acknowledging its sensitive nature.

You couldn't go off to dinner and say 'I've just finished laying out a body'. Who would want to sit next to you.

★★★★★★

If they're in a bowel ward, for want of a better term, and they're conducting bowel wash-outs and . . . anything else along those lines, it would be uncommon I think that the nurse would go to a restaurant and have a discussion about their day's activities. And I think the general public wouldn't appreciate a discussion of those activities either. . . . We don't like to discuss our private bodily functions overtly – the collective 'we' in the general public. We negatively sanction any discussion of those issues as vulgar.

By recognising that their work concerns things which are not acceptable topics for conversation in 'civilised' society, nurses are also acknowledging that they deal with things which are taboo. Taboo topics have much in common with 'dirty' topics because they often amount to the same thing. For example, talk of faeces is not only taboo but also 'dirty'. That which is dirty is often also taboo but taboo topics are not always dirty. Although nurses' work can be seen as dirty work, the dirty work framework is inadequate to the extent that it does not necessarily accommodate work on the taboo. It is, nevertheless, a notion which has arisen within a theoretical framework which contributes to an understanding of the occupation of nursing at the macro level, particularly in the context of occupational statuses and society generally.

NURSES AND THEIR DIRTY WORK

In every culture there are ways of dealing with things that are taboo, as Mary Douglas (1984) has demonstrated and as I discussed in Chapter 3. In our culture, care and assistance with body functions during times of physical incapacity is a role assigned to the nurse.

I think that's a privilege afforded to nurses. It is an expectation of the public that nurses will do that.

******

They [nurses] are expected to do things that are not talked about, not discussed, [that] no-one else sees, and [which] are dirty.

******

I think that's because in the eyes of the general public . . . it's regarded as beneath a person's dignity to deal with other people's excretions, I guess.

Although nurses acknowledge they are assigned this 'dirty' role and that it has a particular social significance, they also notice how some people are uncomfortable about nurses' work and that discomfort is reflected in social encounters outside their work environments. As the data already reported indicate, some people are socially awkward with nurses and they may be embarrassed in nurses' company. Many of the people I interviewed saw this embarrassment and social discomfort as a result of the taboo nature of (some) nurses' work and their dealings with other people's bodies and body products.

I think some people might find it uncomfortable to think about somebody actually nursing a person, doing everything for them. Sometimes I wonder what people think nurses do.

Because some things which nurses do are considered dirty and because they make people feel uncomfortable nurses make provision for it socially. For example, they may not talk about their work in deference to and in recognition of other people's inability to understand it. They are also selective about what they discuss and they sometimes give sanitised accounts of their work when they talk to non-nurses.

I suppose I try to glamorise it a bit, like when I go home I talk about the kind of patients I nursed, whether they were nice, but then I don't talk about that lady peeing on the carpet. I don't mention that, or [patients] spilling their food everywhere.

While nurses acknowledge that their work is often not highly valued and that it makes people feel uncomfortable, they nevertheless regard body care as a crucial element to whatever else their care of patients may involve.

It's always been very important in the sort of work that I've done, for different reasons. In Intensive Care it was because they were sick, and it was very important to them for a wash to be hot. It gave great positive feedback to us because it was well done . . . [and] it showed in its results. It was productive. It induced more rest or more sleep.

Among nurses themselves, there is sometimes a differential value placed on so-called 'basic' (body) care and the more 'technical' aspects of care. This differentiation tends to render some aspects of nursing menial work. Functions which are considered menial and low in status tend to be associated with privatised body functions and it is typical of women's work. Some nurses, however, locate body care in the context of giving comprehensive care and they regard it as an essential part of somological practice. One interviewee described it this way.

I. *I think it [basic body care] is very important in nursing, and I feel that it's something that's often overlooked for the so-called 'more interesting' part of nursing – mainly inexperienced staff who want to to get on and do the more fancy things in nursing and not be bothered with these basic menial jobs.*
R. *But to you it's not basic or menial?*
I. *No, it's part of the patient's care. . . . It's an important part of their care. How can you have a patient that feels comfortable when they are not clean. I suppose it's alright if they're used to living in poor conditions, but most people feel better if they're clean and dry and comfortable.*
R. *So why do you suppose that aspect of nursing is often overlooked?*
I. *Because to some people it's menial. . . . Because [people believe that] everybody can do that, but not everybody can take out sutures and drains . . . or that some people might think that it was dirty.*

What this account illustrates is the apparent ordinariness and simplicity of nurses' work, it highlights the difference between experienced and inexperienced approaches to practice, and it can reflect a taken-for-granted approach to the body which is reflective of wider society. It also shows how nursing can appear to be relatively unskilled and as a consequence it can also be perceived as menial and it can be poorly valued.

In general, the interviewees believed that the privatised and dirty nature of some body functions and taboos about the body contribute to social perceptions of nursing and again it is complicated by the ignorance which surrounds nurses' work.

It's looking after people's bodily fluids, that's the thing. They say 'uh, you have to give out pans all day'. That's what a lot of people interpret that you do, and clean up after anyone who was sick. You know, I haven't given out a pan for ages. . . . A lot of people don't know what you do. That's the big thing.

★★★★★★

They sort of think 'how could they [nurses] do it?', and they don't see the other side to nursing, the parts like talking to patients, making the patient feel better. ... Not many nurses go into it so they can clean up shitty beds. ... A lot of people that I know think that's all you do.

The body care work of nurses, which seems to be so dominant in perceptions of what nurses do as work, is also very closely associated with traditional caring roles assigned to women in our culture. The interviewees believed this was one major factor that contributed to their work being poorly valued – a perceptions which also partly stems from the relative lack of knowledge among the general public about what nurses do as work.

It's a number of things – women's work, a traditional occupation for women, related to caring and nurturing, which is typically female, related to things that women do in the home . . . but a lot of people do not know what nurses do. They conjure up images of the TV where the doctor says 'get me this, get me that' [and the nurse replies] 'yes doctor, no doctor' – images of the doctor's handmaiden.

One of the salient features of nurses' work that closely links it to women's traditional roles is the similarity between body care and mothering.

One of the reasons I guess is that the mother does that for the child, and a woman's work has always been considered menial. So I guess it's associated with that, and it's very basic to everyone's existence.

★★★★★★

I'm sure . . . it's tied up with mothering. I don't think there's any doubt about that. I think it is tied up with the fact that women do it and society sees anything that women do as menial, and body care is traditionally seen as a woman's [role]. You know, if the baby dirties its nappy you call upon the mother, the husband doesn't traditionally do it. . . . It's seen as beneath a man's dignity to deal with vomit, faeces, blood, all of those things, and it is considered OK for a big, strong, macho man to faint at the sight of blood. That's not seen as weak because that's not a man's job anyway. Dealing with body products is a woman's job and beneath a man's dignity . . . and I think that's why men in nursing have had a lot of flack – because they are seen to be doing the menial, body tasks.

Because nursing is so closely tied to traditional women's roles, and in Lewin's (1977:79) view, it 'hovers perilously close', it is easy for it to be ignored, as Oakley (1984) found. The accounts above strongly suggest that considerable ignorance exists about nursing and its occupational functions. Even Elias (1985), who has written about the civilising process, did not mention nurses and their attention to patients in his book, *The Loneliness of the Dying*. To Elias, nurses are invisible.

I wanted to know, from the interviewees, why they thought this should be the case, and why public knowledge of nursing seemed to be so limited. In summary their answers indicated that it was a complex issue which needed to take account, not only of the way the body was dealt with in society, but also the apparently everyday nature of nurses' body care work and the tendency for nurses to conceal or sanitise their work because of those problems of the body. In the process of this concealment, nurses perpetuate public ignorance. They are, to some extent, victims of the work they do and 'the problem of the body'.

They [people] don't really want to know [what nurses do]. . . . People don't understand what nurses do so I guess you don't come freely forward with the information like you would if you said 'I'm a teacher' or 'I'm a bank teller'. . . . We do a lot behind closed doors. We do send the relatives out.

Perhaps the best description of why so much nursing remains invisible, like much of women's work, was provided by a male registered nurse. He saw the problem as one which firmly locates the body at the centre of the cluster of factors which contribute to nurses' identity and public face.

You take someone who has been hospitalised. [They] say 'nurses are wonderful, worth a lot more money'. . . . But I think they would not go home and say 'the nurses were really wonderful, they took really good care of my bowel'. I think they would go home and . . . they wouldn't talk about it. They will talk about 'my operation', 'my doctor', but they won't talk so much about the pan and having the enema and how the nurse did the enema or 'washed me' or all that sort of thing. . . . [It is] soon forgotten and locked away, put away where you don't have to think about it, and they certainly won't talk about it. . . . They go back into a situation where those things aren't talked about. . . . So I think people who have never been hospitalised do not know what nurses do, and even those who have been hospitalised wouldn't tell them.

NURSES' WORK, NURSES' KNOWLEDGE AND A THEORY OF BODY CARE

I have argued in this study that no discipline has yet adequately accommodated the body theoretically, overtly and explicitly because human experience has been subjected to reduction and epistemological fragmentation so that almost every discipline which deals with human experience lays claim to one or other bit. I have also argued that this is a function of what counts as legitimate knowledge, that it is a product of the methods that have been adopted to accumulate knowledge, that the organisation of knowledges militates against a comprehensive understanding of embodied experience, that there has been an emphasis on abstract and reductively derived knowledge, and that practical knowledge has not been systematically studied within mainstream scholarship.

The 'problem of the body', which results, in part, from this fragmentation, originates from the privatised and 'civilised' nature of the body. In effect, the body is associated with, and a source of, things which one does not make public. It is not a topic for legitimate 'normal' social discourse. As such, it is therefore also not a topic for legitimate enquiry.

I have also argued here, though, that nurses accommodate the body in their practice, that they do so in a way which takes account of those things which people have argued are necessary for an adequate understanding of the body, and that they do so every day in their work. Such is the 'problem of the body', however, that nursing is a problematic occupation and discipline. Nursing has an epistemological and methodological crisis with the body. If nursing moves increasingly towards scientising practice, and takes science to mean positivism and reduction, and all that goes with it, nursing will not formally accommodate the body, and neither will any other discipline. If nursing moves toward non-positivist methods to articulate its knowledge it risks continuing as a marginal discipline for as long as science relies so heavily on positivist paradigms.

An understanding of the body can be constructed in a way which is heretical to positivist methodologies and causal models. The data in this study reveal that, while certain trends and patterns can be identified, such as the recovery trajectory, there is considerable variation according to circumstances and personal differences.

To understand the body in social life, and to understand it in nursing in particular, is to have a comprehensive, integrated, composite view of assumed rules (but not necessarily why they exist or where they come from), how those rules influence and structure social relations, how the body as a thing is part of lived experience, and how those notions are integrated into a more general system of social relations. Such knowledge, however, is possible only through experience. Just as we come to be members of a particular culture through experience, so too, we come to be (existentially) human through lived experience of embodiment, and through our experience of what that embodiment means to others. Its meaning to others is integral to our own personal being. Nurses have that understanding of human existence because it is fundamental both to their work and to the knowledge they derive from, and use to guide, practice.

Such is the nature of the way our society deals with the body, however, that nurses' knowledge of the body is not well documented, if it is documented at all, because nurses deal with what people do not **want** to know about. Not only do people not want to know about it, nurses' knowledge of the body has a style and form which to date has not been representative of what has counted as 'proper' knowledge. It is 'practical' knowledge, and as such it is often regarded as the kind of knowledge which does not fit comfortably with theory and research. It is also regarded as the sort of thinking women do – that is, it is perceived as more emotional than rational and not relying heavily on intellect.

The data reported for this study reveal that nurses' knowledge of the body in lived experience and in society generally is anything but irrational and emotional (in the pejorative senses), though it requires control of emotions. It is complex knowledge, and integrative in the context of particular circumstances. It is dependent knowledge because nurses say it 'depends on the person' and 'it depends on the situation'. I have called it *somology* because I wanted a term which would take account of the body (soma), that would include the notion of learning and knowledge (ology) and I wanted the term to be new. I wanted to differentiate it from the term 'holistic', not only because that term has come to mean (too) many things in nursing practice, but because 'holistic' does not adequately summarise the way nurses approach the body in nursing practice.

Nursing is in a unique if not ideal position from which to build a theory of the body, and from which to demonstrate the shortcomings of positivist patterns of enquiry for such an enterprise. Like other areas of women's work, however, nursing has been largely invisible and silent, nurses' knowledge has been poorly investigated, and as an occupation nursing has been minimally understood and poorly valued. The data in this study clearly show that nurses have a vast knowledge of the body and social life – knowledge which is constructed in the context of a society in which people are taught to hide the body and some of its functions. While such a construction of the body continues, there will be social pressure to hide nursing and the work that nurses do, and by virtue of its privatised nature the body will also remain marginal in social science.

References

Abel-Smith B 1977 A history of the nursing profession. Heinemann, London

Ableman P 1982 Anatomy of nakedness. Orbis, London

Ablon J 1984 Little people of America: the social dimensions of dwarfism. Praeger, New York

Albury R M 1987 Babies kept on ice: aspects of Australian press coverage of IVF. Australian Feminist Studies (4): 43–71

Anon. 1986 Stopping sexual harassment: the experts tell you how. RN (Oct): 51–55

Apsler R 1975 Effects of embarrassment on behaviour toward others. Journal of Personality and Social Psychology and Supplement 32 (1): 145–153

Arbeiter J S 1986 Sexual harassment: you can do something about it. RN (Oct): 46–51

Aries P 1985 St Paul and the flesh. In: Aries P, Bejin A (eds) Western sexuality. Basil Blackwell, Oxford

Armstrong D 1983 Political anatomy of the body. Cambridge University Press, Cambridge

Ashley J 1980 Power in structured misogyny: implications for the politics of care. Advances in Nursing Science 2 (3): 3–21

Assey J L, Herbert J M 1983 Who is the seductive patient? American Journal of Nursing (April): 530–532

Barnett K 1972 A theoretical construct of the concepts of touch as they relate to nursing. Nursing Research 21 (2): 102–110

Bart P B, Freeman L, Kimball P 1985 The different worlds of women and men: attitudes toward pornography and responses to 'Not a Love Story' – a film about pornography. Women's Studies International Forum 8 (4): 307–322

Barton E M, Baltes M M, Orzech M J 1980 Etiology of dependence in older nursing home residents during morning care: the role of staff behaviour. Journal of Personality and Social Psychology 38: 423–431

Bates A P 1964 Privacy – a useful concept? Social Forces 42 (May): 429–433

Becker H S, Geer B, Hughes E C, Strauss A 1963 Boys in white: student culture in medical school. University of Chicago Press, Chicago

Beeton I 1987 Mrs Beeton's book of household management. Chancellor Press, London (First published in 1861.)

Bejin A 1985 The decline of the psycho-analyst and the rise of the sexologist. In: Aries P, Bejin A (eds) Western sexuality. Basil Blackwell, Oxford

Benner P 1982a From novice to expert. American Journal of Nursing (March): 402–407

Benner P 1982b Issues in competency-based testing. Nursing Outlook, (May): 303–309

Benner P 1984 From novice to expert. Addison-Wesley, Menlo Park

Benner P, Tanner C 1987 How expert nurses use intuition. American Journal of Nursing (Jan): 23–31

Benner P, Wrubel J 1982 Skilled clinical knowledge: the value of perceptual awareness. Nurse Educator 7 (May/June):11–17

Benner P, Wrubel J 1988 The primacy of caring. Addison-Wesley, Menlo Park

Bennett L 1984 Legal intervention and the female workforce: The Australian Conciliation and Arbitration Court 1907–1921. International Journal of the Sociology of Law 12 (1): 23–36

Berg R 1986 Sexuality: why do women come off second best? In: Grieve N, Burns A (eds) Australian women: new feminist perspectives. Oxford University Press, Melbourne

Bernal E W 1984 Immobility and the self: a clinical-existential inquiry. The Journal of Medicine and Philosophy 9 (1): 75–91

Berry A 1986 Knowledge at one's fingertips. Nursing Times (Dec 3rd): 56–57

Berthelot J M 1986 Sociological discourse and the body. Theory, Culture and Society 3 (3): 155–164

Bhanumanthi P P 1977 Nurses' conceptions of the 'sick role' and 'good patient' behaviour: a cross- cultural comparison. International Nursing Review (Jan/ Feb): 20–24

Birke L, Best S 1980 The tyrannical womb: menstruation and menopause. In: Birke L et al (eds) Alice through the microscope: the power of science over women's lives. Virago, London

Bonawit V, Whittaker Y 1983 The image of nurses and nursing. Australian Nurses Journal 12 (10): 49–54

Brod H 1987 The making of masculinities: the new men's studies. George Allen and Unwin, Sydney

Brodie J A 1984 Response to Dr J. Fawcett's paper. Image: The Journal of Nursing Scholarship XVI (3): 87–89

Buckley T, Gottlieb A (eds) 1988 Blood magic: the anthropology of menstruation. University of California Press, Berkeley

Bullough V L 1972 Sex in history: a virgin field. Journal of Sex Research 8 (2): 101–116

Burbidge G N 1935 Lectures for nurses. Australasian Medical Publishing, Glebe

Buss A H, Iscoe I, Buss E H 1979 Development of embarrassment. Journal of Psychology 103: 227–230

Butler J 1987 Variations on sex and gender: Beauvoir, Wittig and Foucault. In: Benhabib S, Cornell D (eds) Feminism as critique. Polity, Oxford

Caddick A 1986 Feminism and the body. Arena (74): 60–88

Caddick A 1987 Editorial: born of woman, borne of science. Arena (79): 3–8

Caine B, Grosz E A, de Lepervanche M (eds) 1988 Crossing boundaries: feminisms and the critique of knowledges. Allen and Unwin, Sydney

Cameron D, Frazer E. 1987 The lust to kill. Polity Press, Cambridge

Cannon S 1989 Social research in stressful settings: difficulties for the sociologist studying the treatment of breast cancer. Sociology of Health and Illness, 11(1) 62–77

Caplan P (ed) 1987 The cultural construction of sexuality. Tavistock, London

Celermajer D 1987 Submission and rebellion: anorexia and a feminism of the body. Australian Feminist Studies (5): 57–69

Chesler P 1978 About Men. The Women's Press, London

Cohen A 1984 Descartes, consciousness, and depersonalisation: viewing the history of philosophy from a Straussian perspective. Journal of Medicine and Philosophy 9 (1): 7–28

Cohen C H 1986 The feminist sexuality debate: ethics and politics. Hypatia 1 (2): 71–86

Cohen S 1973 Folk devils and moral panic. Paladin, St Albans

Colantonino C 1984 Brandon didn't know his limits. Nursing Life 4 (March/April): 34–35

Colliere M F 1986 Invisible care and invisible women as health care-providers. International Journal of Nursing Studies 23 (2): 95–112

Collins G C, Blodgett D B 1981 Sexual harassment: some see it ... some won't. Harvard Business Review 59 (March/April): 76–93

Colmer M 1979 Whalebone to see-through: a history of body packaging. Jackson and Bacon, London

Connell R W 1983 Which way is up? Essays on sex, class and culture. George Allen and Unwin, North Sydney

Connell R W 1987 Gender and power. George Allen and Unwin, Sydney

Cowles K V 1988 Issues in qualitative research on sensitive topics. Western Journal of Nursing Research 10 (2): 163–179

Creighton H 1987a Sexual harassment: legal implications – Part I. Nursing Management 18 (6): 18, 20, 22

Creighton H 1987b Sexual harassment: legal implications – Part II. Nursing Management 18 (7): 16, 18

Crull P, Cohen M 1984 Expanding the definition of sexual harassment. Occupational Health Nursing (March): 141–145

Davis D S 1984 Good people doing dirty work: a study of social isolation. Symbolic Interaction 7 (2): 233–247

Davis F 1968 Professional socialization as subjective experience: the process of doctrinal conversion among student nurses. In: Becker H S, Geer B, Riesman D, Weiss R S (eds) Institutions and the person. Aldine, Chicago

De La Mare W (no date) Memories of a midget. The New University Society, Edinburgh

de Craemer W 1983 A cross-cultural perspective on personhood. Milbank Memorial Fund Quarterly 61 (1): 19–34

Descartes R 1986 Discourse on method and the meditations. Penguin, Harmondsworth

Dimond R E, Hirt M 1974 Investigation of generalizability of attitudes toward body products as a function of psychopathology and long-term hospitalization. Journal of Clinical Psychology 30 (3): 251–252

Doherty M K, Sirl M B, Ring O I 1965 Modern practical nursing procedures, 11th edn. Dymocks, Sydney

Donnelly G F 1987 The promise of nursing process: an evaluation. Holistic Nursing Practice 1 (3): 1–6

Douglas M 1971 Do dogs laugh? A cross-cultural approach to body symbolism. Journal of Psychosomatic Research 15: 387–390

Douglas M 1984 Purity and danger. Ark Paperbacks, London

Duldt B W 1982 Sexual harassment in nursing, Nursing Outlook 30 (June): 336–343

Dyer R 1985 Male sexuality in the media. In: Metcalf A, Humphries M (eds) The sexuality of men. Pluto, London

Eardley T 1985 Violence and sexuality. In: Metcalf A, Humphries M (eds) The sexuality of men. Pluto, London

Edelmann R J 1981 Embarrassment: The state of research. Current Psychological Review 1: 125–138

Edelmann R J 1985 Social embarrassment: an analysis of the process. Journal of Social and Personal Relationships 2 (2): 195–213

Edelmann R J, Hampson S E. 1979 Changes in nonverbal behaviour during embarrassment. British Journal of Social and Clinical Psychology 18 (Nov): 385–390

Edelmann R J, Hampson S E 1981a The recognition of embarrassment. Personality and Social Psychology Bulletin 7 (1): 109–116

Edelmann R J, Hampson S E 1981b Embarrassment in dyadic interaction. Social Behaviour and Personality 9 (2): 171–177

Edelmann R J, Childs J, Harvey S, Kellock I, Strainclark C 1984 The effect of embarrassment on helping. Journal of Social Psychology 124 (2): 253–254

Ehrenreich B, English D 1976 Witches, midwives and nurses: a history of women healers. Writers and Readers Co-operative, London

Elias N 1978 The civilizing process: the history of manners. Urizen Books, New York (Translated by E. Jephcott.)

Elias N 1985 The loneliness of the dying. Basil Blackwell, Oxford

Elliott C, Kaiser G 1982 Sexual harassment hurts productivity. Modern Healthcare (Sept): 106–107

Ellis H 1913 Studies in the psychology of sex. Vols. 1–6 Davis, Philadelphia

Elshtain J B 1981 Against androgyny. Telos, 47 (Spring): 5–21

Emerson J 1971 Behaviour in private places: sustaining definitions of reality in gynaecological examinations. In: Dreitzel H (ed) Recent Sociology No. 2 Macmillan, London

Emerson R M, Pollner M 1976 Dirty work designations: their features and consequences in a psychiatric setting. Social Problems 23 (3): 243–254

Encyclopedia of Philosophy. 1967 Macmillan and the Free Press, New York

Faberow N L 1963 Taboo topics. Atherton, New York

Fagin C, Diers D 1984 Nursing as metaphor. International Nursing Review.31 (1): 16–17

Fairhurst E 1977 On being a patient in an orthopaedic ward: some thoughts on the definition of the situation. In: Davis A, Horobin B (eds) Medical encounters: the experience of illness and treatment. Croom Helm, London

Faley R H 1982 Sexual harassment: critical review of legal cases with general principles and preventive measures. Personnel Psychology 35 (Autumn) 583–600

Falk P 1985 Corporeality and its fate in history. Acta Sociologica 28 (2): 115–136

Faust B 1980 Women, sex and pornography. Penguin, Harmondsworth

Fawcett J 1984 The metaparadigm of nursing: present status and future refinements. Image: The Journal of Nursing Scholarship XVI (3): 84–86

Featherstone M 1982 The body in consumer culture. Theory, Culture and Society 1 (2): 18–33

Feifel H 1963 Death. In: Faberow N L (ed) Taboo topics. Atherton, New York

Feminist Review (eds) 1987 Sexuality: a reader. Virago, London

Ferguson A 1986 Motherhood and sexuality: some feminist questions. Hypatia 1 (2): 3–22

Field P A, Morse J M 1985 Nursing research: the application of qualitative approaches. Croom Helm, London

Finch J, Groves D (eds) 1983 A labour of love: women, work and caring, Routledge and Kegan Paul, London

Fink E L, Walker B A 1977 Humorous responses to embarrassment Psychological Reports 40 (2): 475–485

Fitzpatrick J, Whall A 1983 Conceptual models of nursing: analysis and application. Brady, Bowie

Flaskerud J, Halloran E 1980 Areas of agreement in nursing theory development. Advances in Nursing Science 3 (1): 1–7

Foss R D, Crenshaw N C 1978 Risk of embarrassment and helping. Social Behaviour and Personality 6 (2): 243–245

Foucault M 1976 The birth of the clinic. Tavistock, London

Foucault M 1984a The archaeology of knowledge. Tavistock, London

Foucault M 1984b The order of things. Tavistock, London

Foucault M 1984c The history of sexuality. Volume I: an introduction.
  Penguin, Harmondsworth
Foucault M 1985a. Discipline and punish. Penguin, Harmondsworth
Foucault M 1985b The battle for chastity. In: Aries P, Bejin A (eds) Western
  sexuality. Basil Blackwell, Oxford
Foucault M 1986b The care of the self. Volume 3 of The history of sexuality.
  Partheon, New York
Foucault M. 1986a The use of pleasure. Volume 2 of The history of sexuality.
  Vintage, New York
Fox R C, Willis D P 1983 Personhood, medicine and American society.
  Milbank Memorial Fund Quarterly 61 (1): 127–147
Freud S 1965 The interpretation of dreams. Avon Books, New York
Freud S 1979a On psycholpathology. Penguin, Harmondsworth
Freud S 1979b Case histories II. Penguin, Harmondsworth
Gadow S 1980 Existential advocacy: philosophical foundation on nursing. In:
  Spicker S F, Gadow S (eds) Nursing: images and ideals. Springer, New York
Gadow S 1982 Body and self: A dialectic. In: Kestenbaum V (ed) The
  humanity of the ill: phenomenological perspectives. University of Tennessee
  Press, Knoxville
Gamarnikow E 1978 Sexual division of labour: the case of nursing. In: Kuhn
  A, Wolpe A M (eds) Feminism and materialism. Routledge and Kegan Paul,
  London
Garfinkel H 1967 Studies in ethnomethodology. Prentice Hall, Engelwood Cliffs
Garvey E G 1987 Life with bodies: an essay. Feminist Studies 13 (2): 409–418
Gatens M 1988 Towards a feminist philosophy of the body. In: Caine B, Grosz
  E A, de Lepervanche M (eds) Crossing boundaries: feminisms and the critique
  of knowledges. Allen and Unwin, Sydney
Genova J 1983 Women and the mismeasure of thought. Hypatia 3 (1): 101–117
Glaser B G, Strauss A L 1965 Awareness of dying. Aldine, Chicago
Glaser B G, Strauss A L 1967 The discovery of grounded theory: strategies for
  qualitative research. Weidenfeld and Nicolson, London
Glaser B G, Strauss A L 1968 Time for dying. Aldine, Chicago
Goffman E 1956 Embarrassment and social organisation. American Journal of
  Sociology 62 (Nov): 264–271
Goffman E 1955 On facework. Psychiatry 18 (August): 213–231
Goffman E 1981 Stigma.: notes on the management of spoiled identity.
  Penguin, Harmondsworth
Gordon C 1980 Michel Foucault: power/knowledge. Harvester, Brighton
Gortner S R 1983 The history and philosophy of nursing science and research.
  Advances in Nursing Science (Jan): 1–8
Greer G 1971 The female eunuch. Paladin, London
Greer G 1987a Lady love your cunt. In: Greer G The madwoman's
  underclothes: essays and occasional writings 1968–85. Picador, London
Greer G 1987b Body odour and the persuaders. In: Greer G The madwoman's
  underclothes: essays and occasional writings 1968–85. Picador, London
Gross F, Stone G 1964 Embarrassment and the analysis of role requirements.
  American Journal of Sociology 70 (1): 1–15
Grosz E 1987 Notes towards a corporeal feminism. Australian Feminist Studies
  (5): 1–16
Gunew S 1987 Male sexuality: feminist interpretations. Australian Feminist
  Studies (5): 71–84
Hacker S S 1984 Students' questions about sexuality: implications for nurse
  educators. Nurse Educator 9 (4): 28–31
Haraway D 1988 Situated knowledges: the science question in feminism and the
  privilege of partial perspective. Feminist Studies 14 (3): 575–599

Harding S. 1984 Is gender a variable in conceptions of rationality? a survey of issues. In: Gould C C (eds) Beyond domination: new perspectives on women and philosophy. Rowman and Allanheld, Totawa

Harding S 1986 The science question in feminism. Cornell University Press, Ithaca

Harre R 1986 Is the body a thing? International Journal of Moral and Social Studies 1 (3): 189–203

Hartmann F 1984 The corporeality of shame: Px and Hx at the bedside. The Journal of Medicine and Philosophy 9 (1): 63–74

Hartsock N C M 1984 Gender and sexuality: masculinity, violence and domination. Humanities in Society 7 (1–2): 19–45

Haug F (ed) 1987 Female sexualization: a collective work of memory. Verso, London

Heath C 1988 Embarrassment and interactional organization. In: Drew P, Wootton A (eds) Erving Goffman: exploring the interaction order. Polity Press, Cambridge

Heinrich K T 1987 Effective responses to sexual harassment. Nursing Outlook 35 (2): 70–72

Henderson V 1964 The nature of nursing. American Journal of Nursing (Aug): 62–68

Henderson V 1982 The nursing process: is the title right? Journal of Advanced Nursing 7: 103–109

Henderson V, Nite G 1978 Principles and practice of nursing, 6th edn. Macmillan, New York

Henley N M 1973 The politics of touch. In: Brown P (ed) Radical psychology. Tavistock, London

Hirt M L, Ross W D, Kurtz R, Gleser G C 1969 Attitudes toward body products among normal subjects. Journal of Abnormal Psychology, 74: 486–489

Hite M 1988 Writing — and reading — the body: female sexuality and recent feminist fiction. Feminist Studies, 14 (1): 121–142

Hite S 1976 The Hite report: a nation-wide study of female sexuality. Macmillan, New York

Hochschild A R 1983 The managed heart: commercialization of human feeling. University of California Press, Berkeley

Hochschild A R 1975 The sociology of feeling and emotion: selected possibilities. In: Millman M, Kanter R M Another voice. Feminist perspectives on social life and social science. Anchor, New York

Hollway W 1987 'I just wanted to kill a woman' Why? The ripper and male sexuality. In: Feminist Review (eds) Sexuality: a reader. Virago, London

Hubbard R 1988 Science, facts, and feminism. Hypatia 3 (1) 5–17

Hughes E 1971 Good people and dirty work. In: The sociological eye: selected papers. Aldine Atherton, Chicago

Humphris M R 1979 The nursing process: an application of scientific method. Australian Nurses Journal 9 (4): 30–31

Hyndman D C 1985 The good go to heaven and the bad go to hell: doing patienthood on the orthopaedic ward. In: Manderson L (ed) Australian ways. Allen and Unwin, Sydney

Irigaray L 1987 Sexual difference. In: Moi T (ed) French feminist thought: a reader. Basil Blackwell, Oxford

Jackson M 1984a Sexology and the social construction of male sexuality (Havelock Ellis). In: Coveney L, Jackson M, Jeffreys S, Kaye L, Mahony P (eds) The sexuality papers. Hutchinson, London

Jackson M 1984b Sexology and the universalization of male sexuality (from Ellis to Kinsey, and Masters and Johnson). In: Coveney L, Jackson M, Jeffreys S, Kaye L, Mahony P (eds) The sexuality papers. Hutchinson, London

Jaggar A M, Bordo S R (ed)1989 Gender/body/knowledge. Rutgers University Press, New Brunswick

Jeffrey R 1979 Normal rubbish: deviant patients in casualty departments. Sociology of Health and Illness 1 (1): 90–107

Jordheim A E 1986 What's the best way to handle a sexually aggressive patient? Journal of Practical Nursing 36 (4): 30–33

Jourard S M 1966 An exploratory study of body accessibility. British Journal of Social and Clinical Psychology 5: 221–231

Jourard S M, Rubin J E 1968 Self-disclosure and touching: a study of two modes of interpersonal encounter and their interaction. Journal of Humanistic Psychology 8: 39–48

Jourard S M 1967 Out of touch: the body taboo. New Society 10 (267): 660–662

Kalisch P A, Kalisch B J 1982a Nurses on prime-time television. American Journal of Nursing (Feb) 264–270

Kalisch P A, Kalisch B J 1982b The image of the nurse in motion pictures. American Journal of Nursing (April) 605–611

Kalisch P A, Kalisch B J 1985 Nursing images: the TV news picture. Nursing Management (April): 39–48

Kalisch P A, Kalisch B J, Clinton J 1982 The world of nursing on prime time television, 1950 to 1980. Nursing Research 31 (6): 358–363

Keat R 1986 The human body in social theory: Reich, Foucault and the repressive hypothesis. Radical Philosophy 42 (Winter/Spring): 24–32

Keller E V 1983 Gender and science. In: Harding S, Hintikka M B (eds) Discovering reality: feminist perspectives on epistemology, metaphysics, methodology, and philosophy of science. Reidel, Dordrecht, Holland

Keller E V 1988 Feminist perspectives on science studies. Thesis Eleven (21): 65–81

Kelly M P 1982 Good and bad patients: a review of the literature and a theoretical critique. Journal of Advanced Nursing 7: 147–156

Kemper T D 1978 Toward a sociology of emotions: some problems and some solutions. The American Sociologist 13 (1): 30–41

Kern S 1975 Anatomy and destiny: a cultural history of the human body. Bobbs-Merrill, Indianapolis

Kinsey A C, Pomeroy W B, Martin C E 1948 Sexual behaviour in the human male. Saunders, Philadelphia

Kinsey A C, Pomeroy W B, Martin C E, Gebhard P H 1953 Sexual behaviour in the human female. Saunders, Philadelphia

Kirby V 1987 On the cutting edge: feminism and clitoridectomy. Australian Feminist Studies (5): 35–55

Knapp P H 1967 Some riddles of riddance: relationships between eliminative processes and emotion. Archives of General Psychiatry 16: 586–602

Kristeva J 1982 Powers of horror: an essay on abjection. Columbia University Press, New York

Kroker A, Kroker M (eds) 1988a Body invaders: sexuality in the postmodern condition. Macmillan, London

Kroker A, Kroker M 1988b Panic sex in America. In: Kroker A, Kroker M (eds) Body invaders: sexuality in the postmodern condition. Macmillan, London

Kubie L S 1937 The fantasy of dirt. Psychoanalytic Quarterly 6: 388–424.

Kuhn T S 1970 The structure of scientific revolutions, 2nd edn. University of Chicago Press, Chicago

Kupfermann J 1979 The MsTaken body. Granada, London

Kurtz R M, Hirt M L, Ross W D, Gleser G, Hertz M A 1968 Investigation of the affective meaning of body products. Journal of Experimental Research in Personality 3: 9–14

La Monica E 1979 The nursing process: a humanistic approach. Addison-Wesley, Menlo Park

Lange L 1983 Woman is not a rational animal: on Aristotle's biology of reproduction. In: Harding S, Hintikka M B (eds) Discovering reality: feminist perspectives on epistemology, metaphysics, methodology, and philosophy of science. Reidel, Dordrecht, Holland

Lawler J 1984 Becoming a nurse educator: the resocialisation of clinically practising general nurses into the role of nurse educator, and the implications this has for nursing as a practice discipline. Master of Education thesis, University of New England, unpublished.

Leach E 1958 Magical hair. Journal of the Royal Anthropological Institute 88: 147–164

Leder D 1984 Medicine and paradigms of embodiment. The Journal of Medicine and Philosophy 9 (1): 29–44

Levin J, Arluke A 1982 Embarrassment and helping behaviour. Psychological Reports 51 (3): 999–1002

Lewin E 1977 Feminist ideology and the meaning of work: the case of nursing. Catalyst (10–11): 78–103

Lloyd G 1984 The man of reason: 'male' and 'female' in western philosophy. Methuen, London

Long D C 1970 The philosophical concept of a human body. In: Spicker S F (ed) The philosophy of the body. Quadrangle, Chicago

Longino H 1988 Science, objectivity, and feminist values. Feminist Studies 14 (3): 561–574

Lorber J 1975 Good patients and problem patients: conformity and deviance in a general hospital. Journal of Health and Social Behaviour 16: 213–225

Loudon J B 1977 On body products. In: Blacking J (ed) The anthropology of the body. Academic Press, London

Lublin J R 1984 A discussion of four evaluative reports on graduates of basic nurse education programs in Colleges of Advanced Education and hospitals: a report to the Commonwealth Tertiary Education Commission Evaluations and Investigations Program. Australian Government Publishing Service, Canberra

Ludbeck E 1987 'A new generation of women': progressive psychiatrists and the hypersexual female. Feminist Studies 13 (3): 513–543

Lynch M 1987 The body: thin is beautiful. Arena (79): 128–145

MacDonald L M, Davies M F 1983 Effects of being observed by a friend or stranger on felt embarrassment and attributions of embarrassment. Journal of Psychology 113 (2): 171–174

Macquarie Dictionary, The 1985 Macquarie Library, Dee Why

Marriner A 1983 The nursing process: a scientific approach to nursing care, 3rd edn. Mosby, St. Louis

Martin E 1987 The woman in the body. Beacon Press, Boston

Masters W H, Johnson V E 1966 Human sexual response. Little Brown, Boston

Matthews J J 1987 Building the body beautiful. Australian Feminist Studies (5): 17–34

Mauksh I G, David M 1972 Prescription for survival. American Journal of Nursing 72 (12): 2189–2193

Mauss M 1973 Techniques of the body. Economy and Society 2 (1): 70–88

McCorkle R 1974 Effects of touch on seriously ill patients. Nursing Research, 23 (2): 125–132

McFarlane J 1976 A charter for caring. Journal of Advanced Nursing 1: 187–196

McHugh M 1986 Nursing process: musings on the method. Holistic Nursing Practice 1 (1): 21–28

McNall S G 1983 Pornography: the structure of domination and the mode of production. Current Perspectives in Social Theory 4: 181–203

Melia K M 1979 A sociological approach to the analysis of nursing work. Journal of Advanced Nursing 4: 57–67

Mendelson R 1983 Sexual harassment. Occupational Health Nursing, 31 (11): 47–49

Merleau-Ponty M 1962 The phenomenology of perception. Routledge and Kegan Paul, London

Metcalf A, Humphries M (eds) 1985 The sexuality of men. Pluto, London

Miller A 1984 Nurse/patient dependency – a review of different approaches with particular reference to studies of the dependency of elderly patients. Journal of Advanced Nursing 9: 479–486

Miller C, Swift K 1976 Words and women. Anchor Press/Doubleday, New York

Modigliani A 1968 Embarrassment and embarrassability Sociometry, 31: 313–326

Modigliani A 1971 Embarrassment, facework, and eye contact: testing a theory of embarrassment. Journal of Personality and Social Psychology 17 (1): 15–24

Montagu A 1978 Touching. The human significance of the skin, 2nd edn. Harper and Row, New York

Moye A 1985 Pornography. In: Metcalf A, Humphries M (eds) The sexuality of men. Pluto, London

Mullins E 1985 The painted witch. Secker and Warburg, London

Munhall P L 1982a Methodological fallacies: a critical self-appraisal. Advances in Nursing Science (July): 41–49

Munhall P L 1982b Nursing philosophy and nursing research: in apposition or opposition? Nursing Research 31 (3): 176–177, 181

Murphy S S 1986 How the victim pays the price. RN (Oct): 48–49

Neklin D 1983 The politics of personhood. Milbank Memorial Fund Quarterly 61 (1): 101–112

Newman S 1984 Anxiety, hospitalization, and surgery. In: Fitzpatrick R, Hinton J, Newman S, Scrambler G (eds) The experience of illness. Tavistock, London

Nightingale F 1969 Notes on nursing. Dover, New York (First published 1859)

O'Neill J 1987 An unhealthy state of affairs. The Sydney Morning Herald Sept. 19th

O'Neill J 1986 Five bodies: the human shape of modern society. Cornell University Press, Ithaca

Oakley A 1974 The sociology of housework. Martin Robertson, Oxford

Oakley A 1981 Interviewing women: a contradiction in terms. In: Roberts H (ed) Doing feminist research. Routledge and Kegan Paul, London

Oakley A 1982 Housewife. Penguin, Harmondsworth

Oakley A 1984 The importance of being a nurse. Nursing Times Dec. 12th: 24–27

Orem D E 1980 Nursing: concepts of practice, 2nd edn. McGraw-Hill, New York

Orr J 1987 Ain't misbehaving? Nursing Times March 4th: 25

Padgug R 1979 Sexual matters: on conceptualising sexuality in history. Radical History Review (20): 3–23

Parker J M 1988 Theoretical perspectives in nursing: from microphysics to hermeneutics. Paper presented at the Third Nursing Research Forum, Lincoln School of Health Science, La Trobe University, Melbourne, March

Parsons T 1951 The social system. Free Press, London

Pelligrino E D, Spiker S F 1984 'Back to the origins': Erwin Strauss – philosopher of medicine, philosopher in medicine. Journal of Medicine and Philosophy 9 (1): 1–5

Perkins R, Bennett G 1985 Being a prostitute. George Allen and Unwin, Sydney

Person E S 1980 Sexuality as the mainstay of identity: psychoanalytic perspectives. Signs: Journal of Women in Culture and Society 5 (4): 605–630

Petchesky R P 1986 Abortion and women's choice. Verso, London

Petronio S 1984 Communication strategies to reduce embarrassment differences between men and women. Western Journal of Speech Communication 48 (1): 28–38

Polhemus T (ed) 1978 Social aspects of the body. Penguin, Harmondsworth

Power M 1975 Women's work is never done - by men. A socio-economic model of sex-typing in occupations. The Journal of Industrial Relations (Sept): 225–239

Reich W 1975 The function of the orgasm. Pocket Books, New York

Reiger K 1987 The embodiment of resistance: reproductive struggles and feminism. Arena (79): 92–107

Rich A 1980 Compulsory heterosexuality and lesbian experience. Signs: Journal of Women in Culture and Society 5 (4): 631–660

Rich R 1986 Feminism and sexuality in the 1980s. Feminist Studies, 12 (3): 525–561

Ridgway B 1984a Sexual harassment. The Lamp 41 (8): 19–21

Ridgway B 1984b The Anti-Discrimination Act and you. The Lamp 41 (9): 22–24

Roberts H E 1977 The exquisite slave: the role of clothes in the making of the Victorian Woman. Signs: Journal of Women in Culture and Society 2 (3): 554–569

Rogers L 1988 Biology, the popular weapon: sex differences in cognitive function. In: Caine B, Grosz E A, de Lepervanche M (eds) Crossing boundaries. Feminisms and the critique of knowledges. Allen and Unwin, Sydney

Ross W D, Hirt M L, Kurtz R 1968 The fantasy of dirt and attitudes towards body products. Journal of Nervous and Mental Disease 146: 303–309

Rothfield P 1986 Subjectivity and the language of the body. Arena (75): 157–165

Ruth S 1987 Bodies and souls/sex, sin and senses in patriarchy: a study in applied dualism. Hypatia 2 (1): 149–163

Sartre J-P circa 1960 Being and nothingness. Philosophical Library, New York

Scarry E 1985 The body in pain: the making and unmaking of the world. Oxford University Press, New York

Scheflen A E 1965 Quasi-courtship behaviour in psychotherapy. Psychiatry 28 (Aug): 245–257

Schutz A 1962 Common sense and scientific interpretation of human action. In: Collected papers I: the problem of social reality. Martinus Nijhoff, The Hague

Schwartz H, Jacobs J 1979 Qualitative Sociology: a method to the madness. Free Press, New York

Scott R 1981 The body as property. Allen Lane, London

Shalom A 1989 The body/mind conceptual framework and the problem of personal identity. Humanities Press International, Atlantic Highlands

Sharrock W, Anderson B 1986 The Ethnomethodologists. Tavistock, London

Shorter E 1984 A history of women's bodies. Penguin, Harmondsworth

Showalter E, Showalter E 1970 Victorian women and menstruation. Victorian Studies XIV (1): 83–89

Silva M C, Rothbart D 1984 An analysis of changing trends in philosophies of science on nursing theory development. Advances in Nursing Science (Jan) 1–13

Smith F B 1971 Ethics and disease in the later nineteenth century: the Contagious Diseases Acts. Historical Studies 15 (57): 118–135

Smith W B, Lew Y L 1975 Nursing care of the patient, 4th edn. Dymocks, Sydney

Spender D 1981 Men's studies modified: the impact of feminism on the academic disciplines. Pergamon Press, Oxford

Spender D 1985 Man made language, 2nd edn. Routledge and Kegan Paul, London

Stannard C I 1973 Old folks and dirty work: the social conditions for patient abuse in a nursing home. Social Problems 20 (3): 329–342

Stockwell F 1984 The unpopular patient. Croom Helm, London

Strang J 1984 Working women: a appealing look at the appalling uses and abuses of the feminine form. Abrams, New York

Strathern M 1985 Dislodging a world view: challenge and counter-challenge in the relationship between feminism and anthropology. Australian Feminist Studies (1): 1–25

Strauss A L 1987 Qualitative analysis for social scientists. Cambridge University Press, Cambridge

Strong P M 1980 Doctors and dirty work — the case of alcoholism. Sociology of Health and Illness 2 (1): 24–47

Suleiman S R (ed) 1986 The female body in western culture. Harvard University Press, Cambridge

Tannahill R 1980 Sex in history. Hamish Hamilton, London

Taylor S E 1979 Hospital patient behaviour. Journal of Social Behaviour 35 (1): 156–184

Tiefer L 1986 In pursuit of the perfect penis: The medicalization of male sexuality. American Behavioural Scientist (May): 579–599

Tinkle M B, Beaton J L 1983 Toward a new view of science: Implications for nursing research. Advances in Nursing Science 6 (1): 27–37

Todd A C 1983 Women's bodies as diseased and deviant: historical and contemporary issues. Research in Law, Deviance and Social Control 5: 83–95

Tuana N 1988a Introduction. Hypatia 3 (1): 1–4

Tuana N 1988b The weaker seed: the sexist bias of reproductive theory. Hypatia 3 (1): 35–59

Turner B S 1982 The governance of the body: medical regimens and the rationalization of the diet. British Journal of Sociology 33: 254–269

Turner B S 1984 The body and society: explorations in social theory. Basil Blackwell, Oxford

Ussher J M 1989 The psychology of the female body. Routledge, London

Vincinus M 1982 Sexuality and power: a review of current work in the history of sexuality. Feminist Studies (Spring): 133–156

Waddington I 1973 The role of the hospital in the development of modern medicine: a sociological analysis. Sociology 7 (2): 211–224

Walby S, Hay A, Soothill K. 1983 The social construction of rape. Theory, Culture and Society 2 (1): 86–98

Warner M 1987 Monuments and maidens: the allegory of the female form. Pan Books, London

Warren C A B 1988 Gender issues in field research. Volume 9 of Qualitative research methods. Sage, Newbury Park

Warren M A 1986 The social construction of sexuality. In: Grieve N, Burns A (eds) Australian women: new feminist perspectives. Oxford University Press, Melbourne

Watson M H 1975 The meaning of touch. Journal of Communication 25 (3): 104–116

Webster D 1985 Medical students' views of the role of the nurse. Nursing Research 34: 313–317

Weeks J 1981 Sex, politics and society: the regulation of sexuality since 1800. Longman, London

Weinberg M S 1968 Embarrassment: its variable and invariable aspects. Social Forces 46 (3): 382–388

Weinberg M S 1965 Sexual modesty, social meanings and the nudist camp. Social Problems 12 (3): 311–318

Weiss S J 1979 The language of touch. Nursing Research 28 (2): 76–79

Williams R S 1984 Ability, dis-ability and rehabilitation: a phenomenological description. Journal of Medicine and Philosophy 9: 93–112

Willis E 1979 Sister Elizabeth Kenny and the evolution of the occupational division of labour in health care. Australian and New Zealand Journal of Sociology 15 (3): 30–38

Willis E 1983 Medical dominance. George Allen and Unwin, Sydney

Wilson D A J, Najman J M 1982 After Nightingale: a preliminary report of work undertaken by nurses in Queensland. The Australian Nurses Journal 12 (4): 31–36

Winstead-Fry P 1980 The scientific method and its impact on holistic health. Advances in Nursing Science 2 (4): 1–7

Wolf Z R 1986a Nurses' work: the sacred and the profane. Holistic Nursing Practice 1 (1): 29–35

Wolf Z R 1986b Nursing rituals in an adult acute care hospital: an ethnography. Ph.D thesis, University of Pennsylvania

Worsley P (ed) 1978 Introducing sociology. Penguin, Harmondsworth

Young I M 1984 Pregnant embodiment: subjectivity and alienation. The Journal of Medicine and Philosophy 9 (1): 45–62

Zita J N 1988 The premenstrual syndrome: dis-easing the female cycle. Hypatia 3 (1): 77–99

Index

Social control (*contd*)
surveillance and, 61, 62, 63
Social rules transgression, 6–7, 10, 30
context construction and, 146,
159–161
embarrassment and, 137–138
interview technique and, 18
protection of patient privacy and,
166
ritualisation of procedures and, 129
sexual expression and, 149,
150–151
Sociology of body, 56, 66, 67, 68
body-self dialectic, 66, 67
'civilised' behaviour and, 73–74
cultural norms and, 71–73
feminism and, 67–68
self-society paradigm and, 66, 67
theoretical aspects, 65–66
Somological approach, **5**, 11, 20, 22,
29, 57, 102, 124, 125, 144,
155, 215–216, 226
basic body care, 146–150, 161–165
concept of embarrassment and, 135
object body-experiential body
integration and, 161–162, 176,
181
protection rule and, 173
recovery trajectory and, 181
Speed, management of embarrassment
and, 123, 143
Sponging/bed bath, 32–33, 119
first experience of, 119, 120–121,
122, 123
male genitals and, 200
modesty rule and, 149
nursing education, procedure and,
124, 125
nursing texts, 40–41, 43–44
Sputum, management of, 173, 174
State, relationship of body to, 60–64
AIDS and, 63–64
panopticism and, 62, 63
social control and, 61, 62
surveillance and, 61, 62–63
Status of patient, 8, 161
Strauss, Erwin, 59
Surveillance, 216
AIDS and, 64
nursing and, 37, 62–63
social control and, 61, 62
Sutcliffe, P. case, 97

Technical nursing, 30–31, 38, 42, 222
Texts, nursing, 38–44, 52

comprehensive/empirically-based,
43–44
language of, 40, 41, 42
nursing procedures, 39–43
object body and, 40, 41
Total patient care, 46
Touch, 107, 110–112, 113
body accessibility to, 108–110, 117
cultural aspects, 109, 110, 117, 118
first experiences in nursing and,
118, 121
genital areas, 199
penis, 121, 199–201
modesty rule and, 149
professional practice and, 111–112
sexual harassment and, 210
strategies for encounters involving, 7
context definition and, 111–112
exclusion of sexual definition of,
196
Turner, 1, 3, 66, 67, 102, 147, 215

Undressing for examination, 111
Uniform, 152–153

Vaginal examination, 111–112, 146
Vomiting, 165, 166–167, 168

Weinberg, 138–139, 140
Wife/attendant role boundaries, 171
Women's work, 24, 30, 44, 49,
223–224, 226, 227
basic body care as, 4, 52–53
biological determinism and, 50–51
as dirty work, 47
language and, 30, 34
scientising of nursing practice and,
35
sexual exploitation and, 213
stereotypes of, 49–50
terminal care and, 187
Wound dressing, 174, 175